Contents

Ophthalmological assessment

Differentials

Diseases

Preface

Rapid Ophthalmology is crafted to offer a concise, clear and accessible overview of ophthalmology. Primarily, the book is aimed at medical students, especially to complement ophthalmology firms and exam revision. It is not designed to be a textbook but rather a source for quickly finding facts about ophthalmology. For example, one could easily have a copy in clinic and look up a disease using a patient's presenting symptoms. Whilst revising for exams the book provides an extremely efficient resource with sections tailored specifically towards differential diagnosis, assessment and OSCE exams.

This book, however, has a value beyond most revision textbooks. It is a book that will not be defunct on the shelves of a junior doctor or even a general practitioner. I have intended this book to be such that it that contains the information needed for the nonspecialist to diagnose, manage and refer those presenting with ophthalmological conditions.

Finally, there is the cohort who desire to pursue ophthalmology as a career. This book would serve that cohort well as they begin to attain knowledge in preparation for a career in ophthalmology.

Zahir Mirza

Acknowledgements

Thank you to Zainab Laftah who authored the two sections, 'Lid lumps, basal cell carcinoma' and 'Lid lumps, other (malignant)'.

Abbreviations

►	Denotes that an urgent referral is required
A&E	Accident and emergency
AAION	Anterior ischaemic optic neuropathy
ACE	Angiotensin converting enzyme
AMD	Age-related macular degeneration
ANA	Anti-nuclear antibody
ANCA	Anti-neutrophil cytoplasmic antibodies
BCC	Basal cell carcinoma
BP	Blood pressure
BRVO	Branch retinal vein occlusion
CADASIL	Cerebral autosomal dominant arteriopathy with subcortical infarcts and leukoencephalopathy
CF	Count fingers visual acuity
CN	Cranial nerve
CNS	Central nervous system
CRAO	Central retinal artery occlusion
CRP	C-reactive protein
CT	Computerised tomography scan
CMV	Cytomegalovirus
CRVO	Central retinal vein occlusion
DM	Diabetes mellitus
dsDNA	Double stranded deoxyribonucleic acid
DVLA	Driver and Vehicle Licensing Agency
ECG	Electrocardiography
ERD	Exudative retinal detachment
ESR	Erythrocyte sedimentation rate
FBC	Full blood count
FFA	Fundus fluorescein angiography
GCA	Giant cell arteritis
GCL	Ganglion cell layer
HAART	Highly active antiretroviral treatment
HLA	Human leukocyte antigens
HM	Hand movements visual acuity
HSV	Herpes simplex virus
HZO	Herpes zoster ophthalmicus
ILM	Inner limiting membrane
IO	Inferior oblique
IOP	Intraocular pressure
IR	Inferior rectus
ITU	Intensive care unit

LR	Lateral rectus
M,C &S	Microscopy culture and sensitivity
MR	Medial rectus
MRA	Magnetic resonance angiography
MRI	Magnetic resonance imaging
NA	Noradrenaline
NFL	Nerve fibre layer
NPL	Nil perception of light visual acuity
NSAIDs	Nonsteroidal anti-inflammatory drugs
NVD	Neovascularization at the disc
NVE	Neovascularization elsewhere
OD	*Omni dei* (once a day)
ONL	Outer nuclear layer
OLL	Outer limiting layer
OSCE	Objective structured clinical examination
PCR	Polymerase chain reaction
PI	Peripheral iridotomy
PL	Perception of light visual acuity
PMR	Polymyalgia rheumatica
PRL	Photoreceptor layer
PVD	Posterior vitreous detachment
RAPD	Relative afferent papillary defect
RF	Rheumatoid factor
ROP	Retinopathy of prematurity
RPE	Retinal pigment epithelium
RRD	Rhegmatogenous retinal detachment
SCC	Squamous cell carcinoma
SO	Superior oblique
SR	Superior rectus
TB	Tuberculosis
TORCH	Toxoplamosis, other, rubella, cytomegalovirus, herpes
TRD	Tractional retinal detachment
U&E	Urea and electrolytes
UV	Ultraviolet
VEGF	Vascular endothelial growth factor
VZV	Varicella-zoster virus

About the companion website

This book is accompanied by a companion website:

 www.wileyrapids.com/ophthalmology

The website contains additional ophthalmic images in PowerPoint format for you to download.

Basic anatomy and physiology

Rapid Ophthalmology, First Edition. Zahir Mirza.
© 2013 John Wiley & Sons, Ltd. Published 2013 by John Wiley & Sons, Ltd.

Note that anatomical layers are described in order from the outer surface of the eye to the inner core.

Osteology of the orbit

ORBITAL FLOOR Maxilla, zygoma, palatine bone.

ORBITAL ROOF Frontal bone, lesser wing of sphenoid.

MEDIAL WALL Maxilla, lacrimal bone, ethmoid, body of sphenoid.

LATERAL WALL Zygomatic bone, greater wing of sphenoid.

Orbital fissures

Superior orbital fissure (Figure 1)

TRANSMITS Lacrimal nerve
Frontal nerve
Trochlear nerve
Superior division of oculomotor nerve
Nasociliary nerve
Inferior division of oculomotor nerve
Abducent nerve

Superior ophthalmic vein
Inferior ophthalmic vein

Inferior orbital fissure

TRANSMITS Infraorbital nerve
Zygomatic nerve
Branches from the pterygopalatine ganglion

Optic canal

TRANSMITS Optic nerve
Ophthalmic artery

The globe

DIMENSIONS Approximate sphere of 2.5 cm diameter
Axial length 24 mm
Volume 5.5 cm^3

LAYERS Superficial to deep: corneoscleral, uveal tract, neural layer.

Cornea (Figure 2)

DIMENSIONS Vertical diameter 10.6 mm
Horizontal diameter 11.7 mm

LAYERS Superficial to deep; corneal epithelium, Bowman's layer, stroma, Descemet's membrane, corneal endothelium.

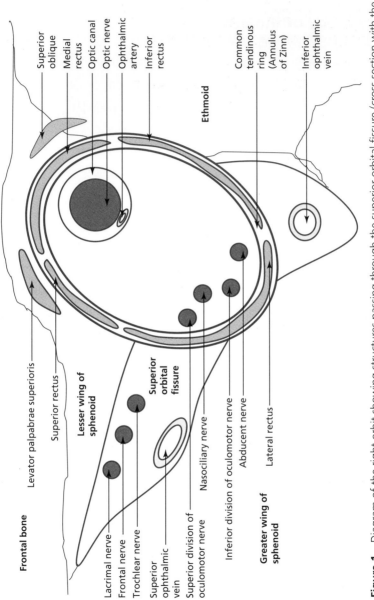
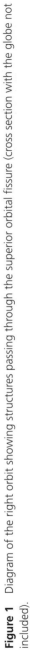

Figure 1 Diagram of the right orbit showing structures passing through the superior orbital fissure (cross section with the globe not included).

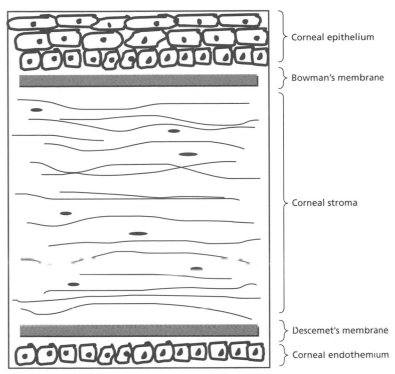

Figure 2   Diagram of a cross-section through the cornea.

SENSORY INNERVATION Ophthalmic division of the trigeminal nerve.

Anatomical terms

ORBITAL SEPTUM Layer of fascia within the eyelids arising from the periosteum of the orbital rim.

LIMBUS Junction between cornea and sclera.

UVEAL TRACT Comprises the iris, ciliary body and choroid.

CHOROID Vascular connective tissue between the sclera and retina. It nourishes the outer third of the retinal. The fovea is dependent on this blood supply for nourishment.

ANTERIOR SEGMENT Portion of the eye between the cornea and the anterior surface of the vitreous humour.

POSTERIOR SEGMENT Posterior two-thirds of the eye that contains the vitreous humour, optic disc, retina, most of the sclera and choroid.

ANTERIOR CHAMBER Formed by the cornea anteriorly and the iris posteriorly.

POSTERIOR CHAMBER Formed by the iris anteriorly and the lens posteriorly.

MACULA LUTEA Yellow area at the centre of the posterior retina that gives rise to fine vision owing to a high concentration of cone receptors.

FOVEA CENTRALIS A depression within the centre of the macula; it provides the most distinct vision as it has the highest density of cone receptors. Inner retinal layers are displaced laterally, hence the depression.

OPTIC DISC The optic nerve and central retinal vessels enter and leave the globe at this site. There are no photoreceptors at the optic disc, hence there is no visual perception of light falling onto this region. Therefore this area gives rise to the blind spot.

Retinal overview

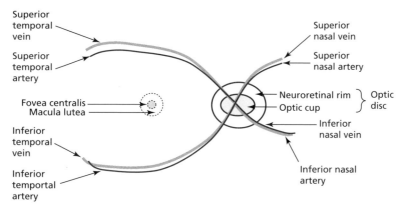

Figure 3   Schematic diagram showing clinical terms used to describe regions of the retina.

Layers of the retina

Lying on the retinal pigment epithelium (RPE) are three cell types in series that form the neurosensory retina; photoreceptive rods and cones, interneurones and ganglion cells. The RPE provides physiological support to the overlying neurosensory retina. The neurosensory retina converts light to neural impulses.

Figure 4 is a picture, obtained from ocular coherence tomography, that shows almost histological anatomical detail of retinal layers.

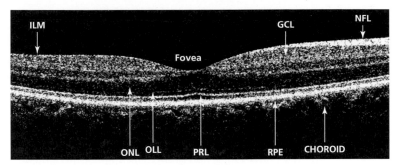

Figure 4   Ocular coherence tomography scan of the retina.
RPE – retinal pigment epithelium (and Bruch's membrane); PRL – photoreceptor layer; OLL – outer limiting layer; ONL – outer nuclear layer; GCL – ganglion cell layer; NFL – nerve fibre layer; ILM – inner limiting membrane.

Blood supply to the eye

Branches of the ophthalmic artery, which is the first cavernous branch of the internal carotid artery, supply the eye (important branches listed below):

Central retinal artery – supplies the inner two-thirds of the retina; however, there are no capillaries from branches of this artery supplying the fovea.
Short posterior ciliary arteries – supply the choroid.
Long posterior ciliary arteries – supply the iris and ciliary body.
Lacrimal artery – supplies lacrimal gland and eyelids.

Ciliary body and lens

This structure joins the choroid to the iris and features specialized surface folds (ciliary processes) that secrete aqueous humour. Through fine filaments (zonules) it supports the lens. Contraction of the ciliary body's muscular component relaxes the zonules and causes the lens to assume a more convex shape and thus allows focusing for near vision (accommodation). The lens is a transparent structure contained in an elastic capsular membrane located posterior to the pupil and iris and anterior to the vitreous.

Trabecular meshwork

Located within the angle between the cornea and iris, this structure is responsible for draining 90% of the aqueous fluid.

Aqueous humour flow

Aqueous humour flows from the posterior chamber, through the pupil and into the anterior chamber. It is taken up by the trabecular meshwork which drains aqueous filled vacuoles into a collecting channel known as Schlemm's canal. These drain into the vortex veins that contribute to the venous drainage of the eye.

Tears
Every blink recreates a three-layer tear film that coats the ocular surface.
From anterior to posterior:

Lipid (from eyelid Meibomian glands)
Aqueous (from the lacrimal gland and accessory conjunctival lacrimal glands)
Mucin (from conjunctival Goblet cells)

Vitreous humour
The transparent gel-like substance that occupies the posterior segment of the eye. It is composed 99% of water with collagen, hyaluronic acid and other proteins forming the remainder.

Ocular muscles (origin / insertion / primary actions [Figure 5])
Superior rectus (SR)
Origin – common tendinous ring
Insertion – sclera
Innervation – cranial nerve III (superior division)
Primary action – elevation of the globe

Inferior rectus (IR)
Origin – common tendinous ring
Insertion – sclera
Innervation – cranial nerve III (inferior division)
Primary action – depression of the globe

Medial rectus (MR)
Origin – common tendinous ring
Insertion – sclera
Innervation – cranial nerve III (inferior division)
Primary action – adduction

Lateral rectus (LR)
Origin – common tendinous ring
Insertion – sclera
Innervation – cranial nerve VI
Primary action – abduction

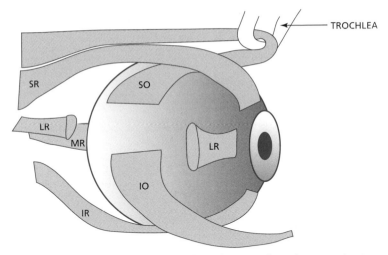

Figure 5 Schematic diagram using a lateral view to show the approximate insertions of extraocular muscles onto the globe. Note that a portion of the lateral rectus has been removed in this diagram in order to show the insertions of the oblique muscles. Also, the medial rectus inserts onto the medial aspect of the globe thus its insertion cannot be visualized from this view.

Superior oblique (SO)
Origin – sphenoid bone; however, its functional origin is from the trochlea which acts like a pully
Insertion – sclera
Innervation – cranial nerve IV
Primary action – intorsion (the secondary action is depression, especially in the adducted position)

Inferior oblique (IO)
Origin – anterior orbital floor
Insertion – sclera
Innervation – cranial nerve III (inferior division)
Primary action – extorsion (the secondary action is elevation in adduction)

The visual pathway (Figures 6 and 7)
The nasal retinal receives light from the temporal visual field and the temporal retina receives light from the nasal visual field. Photoreceptors within the retina act as the first-order neurones in the visual pathway. These then synapse with bipolar cells (second-order neurones) which synapse with ganglion cells (third-order neurones). The optic nerve contains axons from these ganglion cells.

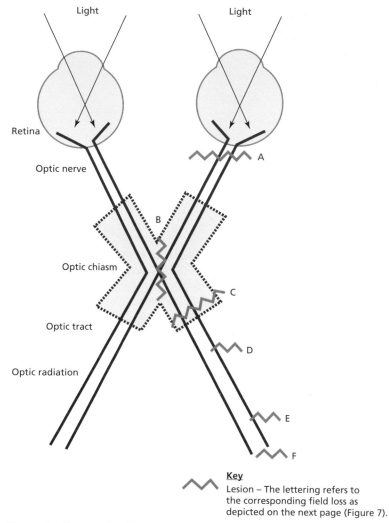

Figure 6   The visual pathway.

The fibres of the optic nerve converge at the optic chiasm and here fibres from the nasal retina cross over. Fibres from the temporal retina remain uncrossed. The optic tracts commence posterior to the chiasm and connect to the lateral geniculate body.

The axons of the lateral geniculate body travel via the optic radiations in the temporal and parietal lobes to the primary visual cortex in the occipital lobe.

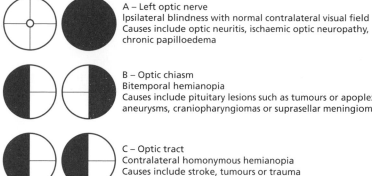

A – Left optic nerve
Ipsilateral blindness with normal contralateral visual field
Causes include optic neuritis, ischaemic optic neuropathy, chronic papilloedema

B – Optic chiasm
Bitemporal hemianopia
Causes include pituitary lesions such as tumours or apoplexy, aneurysms, craniopharyngiomas or suprasellar meningioma

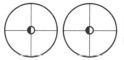

C – Optic tract
Contralateral homonymous hemianopia
Causes include stroke, tumours or trauma

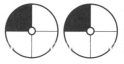

D – Optic radiation – temporal lobe
Superior quadrantanopia – This would correspond to a lesion in the anterior and inferior loops of the optic radiation in the temporal lobe. These areas may be affected by tumours, infection or vascular lesions

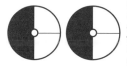

E – Optic radiation – Posterior pariatal and occipital lobe
Homonymous hemianopia with macular sparing. Posterior cerebral artery occlusion with occipital infarction may spare the macular due to its large representation in the occipital lobe or due to collateral blood supply to the areas representing the macular

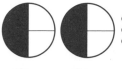

F – Tip of the occipital lobe
Homonymous hemianopic scotomas caused, for example, by a lesion of the tip of the occipital lobe

Note, lesions are described as if affecting the left side as shown in Figure 6.

Figure 7   Visual field defects.

Pupillary reflexes
Direct and consensual light reflex
Pathway: uniocular light stimulus – retinal stimulation – optic nerve – ipsilateral pretectal nucleus – bilateral sympathetic nuclei of cranial nerve (CN) III (Edinger-Westphal) – CN III (via ciliary ganglion) – iris sphinter pupillae muscles of each eye – bilateral pupil constriction (miosis)

Accommodation
Pathway: change in fixation from a distant target to near – retinal stimulation – optic nerve – visual cortex – descending fibres from cortex – then fibres travel through one of two pathways:

(a) most fibres travel to cause convergence; internal capsule –
    midbrain – oculomotor nuclei – oculomotor nerve to medial recti –
    both medial recti contract – convergence of visual axes;
(b) some synapse bilaterally with Edinger-Westphal nuclei
    (parasympathetic fibres) – CN III (via ciliary ganglion) – ciliary muscle
    (causing the lens to assume a more convex shape with greater
    refractive power) and iris sphincter pupillae muscles of each eye
    (causing bilateral pupil constriction).

Pupil defects
Holmes-Adie pupil
A mid-dilated pupil with very slow reaction to light and a normal or
slow reaction to accommodation. Recovery from constriction is slow. It
is unilateral in 80% of cases but can progress to become bilateral thus
mimicking Argyll Robertson pupils. It typically affects young women.
Holmes-Adie syndrome features these findings in association with
absent knee/ankle jerk.

Essential anisocoria
This is sometimes referred to as 'physiological anisicoria'. The pupils are
of a different size but all pupil reactions are normal. It is estimated that
20% of the normal population have pupils of a different size with no
underlying pathological cause.

Argyll Robertson pupils
Both pupils are small and irregular pupils. They react to
accommodation but not to light and are found in neurosyphilis and
diabetic autonomic neuropathy.

Horner's syndrome
A Miotic pupil with 2 mm of ptosis and unilateral anhydrosis of the
upper face (see Horner's syndrome, below, **p. 85**).

Cranial nerve III palsy (complete)
Fixed and dilated pupil with ptosis and an eye that is abducted and
depressed (down and out).

Relative afferent pupillary defect (RAPD) or Marcus Gunn pupil
Following direct stimulation of a pupil by light, both pupils constrict in
normal eyes. In the presence of a relative afferent papillary defect the
following sequence would be observed:

1. Light shone on the normal pupil – constriction of both pupils.

2. Light then swung on to abnormal pupil – dilation of the (abnormal) pupil onto which the light is being shone (and simultaneous dilatation of the normal pupil).

A RAPD indicates a reduction in the afferent input from the retina of the abnormal eye compared to the normal eye because of an optic nerve defect in the former. There may be no RAPD if the optic nerves are equally abnormal.

Myopia, hypermetropia and astigmatism

Emmetropia
Light is brought to focus at the fovea

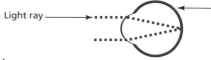

Myopia
Light is brought to focus in front of the fovea

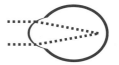

A concave diverging lens will correct myopia

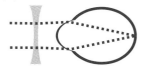

Hypermetropia
Light is brought to focus in behind fovea

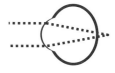

A convex converging lens will correct hypermetropia

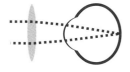

Regular astigmatism
The refractive power of the eye varies due to unequal curvature of a refractive surface. The axes of greatest and least refractive power are at 90 degrees to each other. Often this is due to a compressed corneal shape (sometimes described as a rugby ball shaped cornea).

A toric lens will correct regular astigmatism

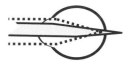

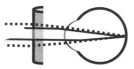

Irregular astigmatism
An irregularly shaped cornea focuses light at various different points and the axis of greatest and least focussing power are not at 90 degrees to each other.

Soft contact lenses cannot correct irregular astigmatism. A rigid contact lens will correct irregular astigmatism by 'replacing' the corneal surface.

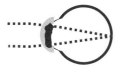

Figure 8   Refractive errors.

Ophthalmological assessment

Rapid Ophthalmology, First Edition. Zahir Mirza.
© 2013 John Wiley & Sons, Ltd. Published 2013 by John Wiley & Sons, Ltd.

History taking

Obtaining an ophthalmic history does not differ in approach from obtaining a history of other systems, i.e. ensuring that a comprehensive analysis of the presenting complaint and associated symptoms is elicited. Side or sides affected (laterality), time course and periodicity are particularity important features. Specific ocular symptoms that one should elicit include:

- visual disturbance
- pain
- floaters
- flashing lights
- halos
- visual field loss
- diplopia.

Past ocular history is an additional and useful component of an ophthalmic history and should include the following:

- contact lens wear
- glasses wear
- ocular/head injury
- ocular surgery
- lazy eye / squints / patching of the eye as a child.

Examination

Examination of the eye should proceed in a methodical manner with focused attention as appropriate.

1. Visual acuity (see OSCE section).
2. Colour vision.
3. Eye movements / diplopia.
4. Visual fields.
5. Pupil reflexes.
6. General and external eye appearance including eyelids e.g. ectropion, entropion, skin laxity, scars, evidence of trauma.
7. Conjunctiva, e.g. colour, blood vessel injection, swelling/oedema (chemosis).
8. Cornea, e.g. clarity (should be stained with fluorescein and examined under a cobalt blue light for epithelial defects).
9. Anterior chamber (typically examined with slit lamp but with pen torch, fluid level may be apparent, e.g. hypopyon = collection of protein/white cells or hyphaema = collection of red blood cells).
10. Pupil size, shape, symmetry and reflexes.

11. Direct ophthalmoscope (see OSCE section):
    Red reflex to check for lens opacity
    Fundus examination.

Also consider trigeminal nerve assessment (in particular corneal sensation) and function of the facial nerve (eye closure).

Examination techniques
Colour vision
A simple check for optic nerve damage can be using a bright red target and asking the patient to comment on the appearance of the target with each eye. Impaired perception of the colour/brightness of the red target, or red desaturation, can indicate early optic nerve pathology.

Ishihara test plates are designed to test for congenital red-green colour blindness. The plates are presented individually to each eye and the patient asked to read the number represented by coloured dots on each plate. The first plate is one that everyone with moderately good visual acuity should be able to read. Inability to read numbers on certain plates are then recorded as these can represent colour vision defects as indicated by a key included with the test.

As optic nerve damage can impair red–green colour vision the test can also be used to detect such pathology.

Pupil reflexes
1. Comment on pupil size and symmetry.
2. Ask the patient to focus on a distant target.
3. Hold an object at about 15 cm from the patient's eyes, ask them to focus on the object and observe for pupil constriction (accommodation).
4. Ask the patient to fixate again on a distant target.
5. Shine the beam of a bright pen torch onto one pupil. Observe that pupil for constriction (direct light reflex).
6. Repeat the process whilst observing the pupil opposite to which the light is being shone (consensual light reflex).
7. Now shine the beam into the other pupil and elicit direct and consensual reflexes.
8. The swinging light test (to test for a relative afferent papillary defect) – the light beam is shone from one pupil and then to the other and back again. The pupil on to which the light beam is swung over to is observed for paradoxical dilatation.

Visual fields by confrontation
The normal visual field extends approximately 60 degrees nasally and 110 degrees temporally. Superior and inferior fields extend 60 degrees and 75 degrees respectively.

Gross defects can be revealed by one of the following clinical examination techniques. These all involve a comparison between the visual field of the patient and the examiner.

The patient is seated at arm's length, in front of the examiner, with the eyes of the patient and examiner on the same horizontal plane.

To test the right eye's visual field the patient is asked to cover their left eye and stare at a static point, for example, the bridge of the nose of the examiner. The examiner closes his right eye so that the visual field of the patient can be approximately compared to his own.

The examiner then holds up either one finger or two fingers, in a quadrant of the peripheral visual field. The patient is then asked how many fingers are being held up. Each quadrant is tested this way. If the responses are correct then the field is deemed to be normal in quadrants tested.

The examiner must continually monitor the patient to ensure that the patient is not deviating their gaze from the specified target (the bridge of the nose in this example). If the patient does look directly at the fingers being held up then inadvertently the central, not the peripheral, visual field would be tested.

An alternative method involves the examiner slowly bringing in the tip of his finger from each peripheral quadrant. The finger should be brought inwards, from outside of the field of view of both the patient and examiner, and towards a central point. The patient is asked to say 'yes' when the tip of the finger first comes into view.

A further possible method involves using a hatpin. A white hatpin can be brought in from the periphery by the examiner instead of a finger. A red hatpin can then be used to map out the patient's blind spot and its size compared to the examiner's own blind spot.

Whichever test is used, the other eye must also be tested in a similar manner, with the contralateral eye covered. Thus when examining the visual field of the patient's left eye, the patient's right eye must be covered and the examiner's left eye must be covered.

Eye movements

When examining eye movements a history of double vision should elicited.

There are various aspects of eye movements assessment.

1. Is there a head tilt or turn?
2. Is there any obvious eso/exo deviation?
3. Eye movements: the patient is asked to follow a target, such as a pen torch, held by the examiner. A suitable instruction may be:

   'Look at the tip of my pen, follow it with your eyes, keeping your head still and letting me know if any time you see double or feel pain.'

Right eye   Left eye

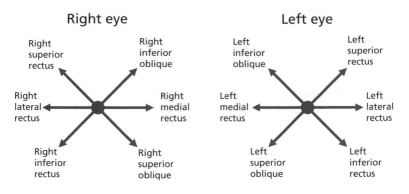

Arrows represent direction of gaze being tested and the names of the main muscle responsible for that movement

Figure 9 Testing eye movements.

The pen is then moved from the centre to peripheral positions whilst both eyes are observed for any abnormalities, such as restriction, nystagmus, double vision, and pain. If there is double vision a check should be made to elicit if this is monocular or binocular diplopia. If diplopia persists after covering one eye, this is monocular diplopia and suggests an underlying refractive cause.

Some prefer to check eye movements by drawing an H pattern with their target whilst ophthalmologists frequently use a 'star pattern' which enables the eye movements in each cardinal direction of gaze to be examined. The latter is depicted in Figure 9 with the corresponding name of the muscle responsible for each of the cardinal movements. The arrows also represent the directions that the target should be moved in when testing eye movements if using a 'star pattern'.

Objective structured clinical examination (OSCE) section
Visual acuity

Testing visual acuity properly requires a standard Snellen chart, an eye occluder and pin hole. Reading or near vision can be tested using specialist charts and is not covered here.

SCHEMA FOR EXAMINATION

- Hand washing
- Introduction
- Explanation of the procedure and consent

> 'I have been asked to test your vision; it will involve testing one eye at a time and you reading some letters on a chart. Is that OK?'

- A Snellen chart is designed to be used at a distance of 6 metres from the patient and is normally backlit. The patient should be placed so that they are 6 metres from the chart. They should wear their normal distance glasses or contact lenses for the test and it should be documented if vision was tested whilst these were being worn.
- One eye is occluded and the patient asked to read down the chart. If the patient can read more than 50% of a line then visual acuity can be recorded as at that line. The distance that the patient is away from the chart is written on the top of the 'fraction' and the line which they can read is recorded below the 'fraction', e.g. if a patient can read the '36' line at 6 metres then visual acuity should be recorded as 6/36 in that eye.
- If the patient achieves normal vision, 6/6 or better, then the test can proceed to the other eye. If not, the following schema should be followed for the eye before testing the other eye.
- If normal vision is not attained, then the vision should be tested with the patient looking through a pinhole. This will reduce the adverse effect of a simple refractive error and may give a better indication of potential visual acuity. For example, a glasses wearer may have extremely poor vision when tested on the Snellen chart if tested without their glasses (unaided) and this would be misleading.
- If the patient cannot read the top line of the chart (i.e. vision is worse than 6/60) then the chart can be brought closer, for example to 1 meter. This new distance must be recorded at the top of the 'fraction',e.g. if the top line of the chart can be read at 1 meter then visual acuity can be recorded at 1/60.
- If a patient can still not read the letters, then the patient can be asked if they can count fingers (CF). The distance at which this is possible is recorded.
- If a patient cannot count fingers, they should be asked to detect hand movements (HM).
- If they cannot detect hand movements, they should be asked to see if they can detect the light of a bright pen torch (PL).
- If not, visual acuity can be recorded as nil perception of light (NPL).

Ophthalmoscopy

This is a skill that is often examined at OSCE examinations. It is most likely that a dummy head with a slide that represents the fundus is used. This should not deter the candidate from regarding the head as though it were a real patient.

SCHEMA FOR EXAMINATION

- Hand washing
- Introduction

- Explanation of the procedure and consent:

  'I have been asked to examine your eyes, this will involve shining a bright light into your eyes, and coming quite close which may mean I need to bring my hand to your forehead. Is that OK?'

- Reduce room illumination and check function of ophthalmoscope. Set focus wheel (typically at zero).
- Hold the ophthalmoscope in the right hand to examine the right eye.
- Ask the patient to fix on a distant target, examine with your right eye.
- From an arm's length, examine for the red reflex and comment on its appearance in both eyes.
- Approach the patient's right eye from a supero-temporal angle, keeping the red reflex in view and get close.
- Ensure full focus of the retinal vessels by adjusting the focusing wheel as appropriate.
- Examine the general appearance of the fundus, vessels, optic disc. Then ask the patient to look at the light so the macula is brought into view. Be prepared to make a comment on each aspect.
- Move on to examine the left eye, holding the ophthalmoscope in the left hand, using your left eye to examine the patient's left eye and repeat the examination of the fundus.
- Thank the patient.
- Collect your thoughts and systematically present your findings and conclusion to the examiner.

Differentials

Rapid Ophthalmology, First Edition. Zahir Mirza.
© 2013 John Wiley & Sons, Ltd. Published 2013 by John Wiley & Sons, Ltd.

Watery eye
Conjunctivitis (especially viral and allergic)
Corneal abrasion
Trauma
Foreign body
Dry eye
Blepharitis
Nasolacrimal duct obstruction
Trichiasis/entropion/ectropion

Proptosis
Thyroid eye disease is the most common cause of unilateral and
bilateral proptosis. Protrusion of the globe due to thyroid eye disease is
more accurately termed exophthalmos.
Orbital cellulitis
Neoplasm
Wegener's granulomatosis
Orbital haemorrhage (secondary to trauma/surgery)
Orbital trauma
Vascular malformations
Sinus mucocoele
Orbital floor fractures (may cause an eye to become enophthalmic,
creating the appearance of the contralateral normal eye appearing
proptosed)

Optic disc atrophy
Glaucoma
Ischaemic optic neuropathy
Central retinal vein/artery occlusion
Papilloedema (chronic)
Optic neuritis (chronic)
Optic nerve compression
Optic neuropathy (traumatic/metabolic/toxic)
Leber's hereditary optic neuropathy

Toxic optic neuropathy
Tobacco
Alcohol
Ethambutol
Amioderone
Isoniazid
Systemic chloramphenicol
Hydroxychloroquine
Lead

Swollen optic discs
Papilloedema – bilaterally swollen discs secondary to raised intracranial pressure (note that swelling may be not be symmetrical and therefore this may *appear* as a unilateral swollen optic disc)
Optic disc drusen
Optic neuritis
Ischaemic optic neuropathy
Central retinal vein occlusion
Grade 4 hypertensive retinopathy
Neoplasm
Inflammatory disease such as sarcoidosis
Thyroid eye disease with optic neuropathy

Ptosis
Cranial nerve III palsy
Myasthenia gravis
Horner syndrome
Trauma
Orbital malignancy
Eyelid inflammation/lump/tumour
Age related

The red eye
Classic presentations of a red eye and associated conditions
BLEPHARITIS Inflammation of the eyelid margins, causing gritty, dry and mildly red eyes.

PRESEPTAL CELLULITIS Swelling and erythema of the eyelid without systemic upset or other features of orbital cellulites.

ORBITAL CELLULITIS Swelling and erythema of the eyelid, systemic upset, fever, difficulty opening the eye, diplopia, proptosis and pain.

CONJUNCTIVITIS Presenting with a red inflamed conjunctiva. Can be due to an allergic, viral or bacterial cause. Vision normal, Photophobia rare.

SUBCONJUNCTIVAL HAEMORRHAGE Painless but dramatic looking well-defined redness of the eye. May or may not be associated with trauma. Vision normal, no photophobia.

KERATITIS Affecting the cornea with circumcorneal vascular injection. Typically significant pain or foreign body sensation with photophobia and variable visual loss.

CORNEAL ABRASION Patients present with acute pain, photophobia and increased tear production. Most are associated with trauma, such as a scratch from a finger nail or from a foreign body.

ANTERIOR UVEITIS (IRITIS) Pain, blurred vision, photophobia, ipsilateral small pupil (miosis) and circumcorneal injection. May be associated with inflammatory conditions such as sarcoidosis or juvenile idiopathic arthritis.

EPISCLERITIS Typically sectorial tender redness with limited ache. Vision normal, no photophobia.

SCLERITIS Severe 'boring' pain/ache of the eye, dramatic dilation of the scleral vessels. Associated with systemic disease such as rheumatoid arthritis.

ACUTE ANGLE CLOSURE GLAUCOMA Severe eye pain, the appearance of halos around lights, nausea/vomiting. A fixed and dilated oval pupil, ciliary injection and raised intraocular pressure.

Differentials – classified anatomically (from anterior to posterior)
EYELIDS Blepharitis
       Preseptal cellulitis
       Orbital cellulitis

CONJUNCTIVA Conjunctivitis
       Subconjunctival haemorrhage

CORNEA Keratitis
       Corneal abrasion

EPISCLERA Episcleritis

SCLERA Scleritis

UVEAL TRACT Anterior uveitis

Differential flow charts
Please see following pages

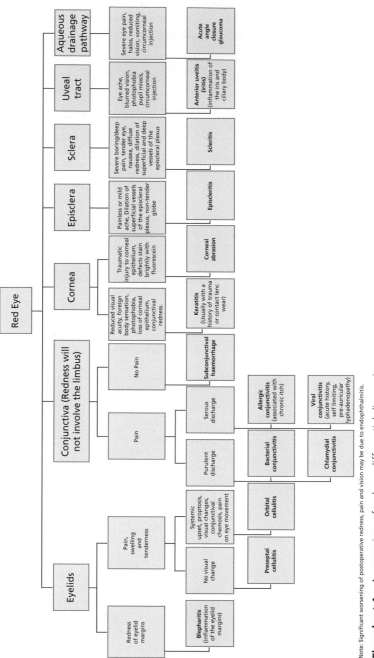

Note: Significant worsening of postoperative redness, pain and vision may be due to endophthalmitis.

Flowchart 1 An overview of red eye differential diagnosis.

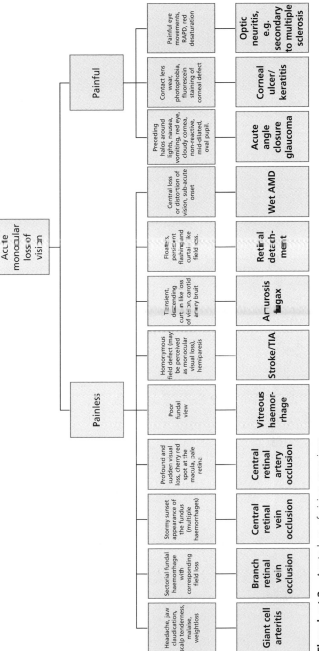

Flowchart 2 Acute loss of vision overview.

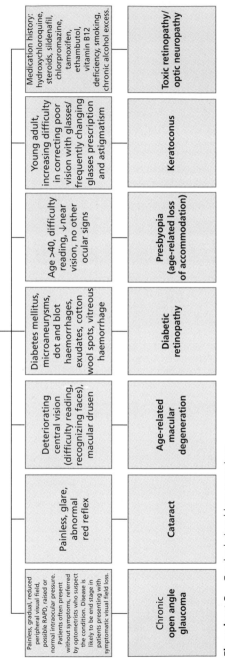

Flowchart 3 Gradual visual loss overview.

Gradual loss of vision

- Painless, gradual, reduced peripheral visual field, possible RAPD, raised or normal intraocular pressure. Patients often present without symptoms, referred by optometrists who suspect the condition. Disease is likely to be end stage in patients presenting with symptomatic visual field loss.
  → **Chronic open angle glaucoma**

- Painless, glare, abnormal red reflex
  → **Cataract**

- Deteriorating central vision (difficulty reading, recognizing faces), macular drusen
  → **Age-related macular degeneration**

- Diabetes mellitus, microaneurysms, dot and blot haemorrhages, exudates, cotton wool spots, vitreous haemorrhage
  → **Diabetic retinopathy**

- Age >40, difficulty reading, ↓ near vision, no other ocular signs
  → **Presbyopia (age-related loss of accommodation)**

- Young adult, increasing difficulty in correcting poor vision with glasses/ frequently changing glasses prescription and astigmatism
  → **Keratoconus**

- Medication history: hydroxychloroquine, steroids, sildenafil, chlorpromazine, tamoxifen, ethambutol, vitamin B12 deficiency, smoking, chronic alcohol excess.
  → **Toxic retinopathy/ optic neuropathy**

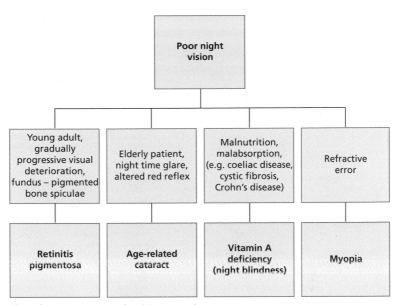

Flowchart 4   Poor night vision overview.

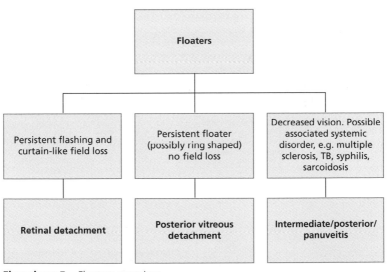

Flowchart 5   Floaters overview.

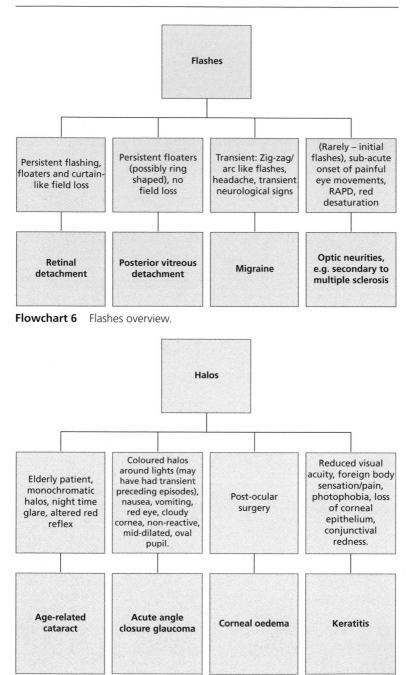

Flowchart 6   Flashes overview.

Flowchart 7   Halos overview.

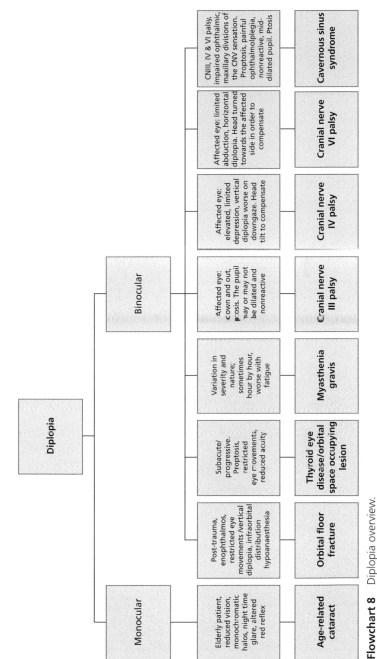

Flowchart 8 Diplopia overview.

Diplopia

Monocular
- Elderly patient, reduced vision, monochromatic halos, night time glare, altered red reflex → **Age-related cataract**

Binocular
- Post-trauma, enophthalmos, restricted eye movements/vertical diplopia, infraorbital distribution hypoanaesthesia → **Orbital floor fracture**
- Subacute/progressive. Proptosis, restricted eye movements, reduced acuity → **Thyroid eye disease/orbital space occupying lesion**
- Variation in severity and nature; sometimes hour by hour, worse with fatigue → **Myasthenia gravis**
- Affected eye: down and out, ptosis. The pupil may or may not be dilated and nonreactive → **Cranial nerve III palsy**
- Affected eye: elevated, limited depression, vertical diplopia worse on downgaze. Head tilt to compensate → **Cranial nerve IV palsy**
- Affected eye: limited abduction, horizontal diplopia. Head turned towards the affected side in order to compensate → **Cranial nerve VI palsy**
- CNIII, IV & VI palsy, impaired ophthalmic, maxillary divisions of the CNV sensation. Proptosis, painful ophthalmolplegia, nonreactive, mid-dilated pupil. Ptosis → **Cavernous sinus syndrome**

Diseases

Rapid Ophthalmology, First Edition. Zahir Mirza.
© 2013 John Wiley & Sons, Ltd. Published 2013 by John Wiley & Sons, Ltd.

Age-related macular degeneration (AMD), dry

DEFINITION Blinding degeneration of the macula characterized by drusen and changes to the retinal pigment epithelium (RPE).

AETIOLOGY Unknown, likely multifactorial. See Associations/risk factors.

ASSOCIATIONS/RISK FACTORS Increased age, female gender (most likely due to increased ages of survival), smoking, hypermetropia, hypertension, race (greater in Caucasians than Blacks), excessive alcohol intake. Cumulative UV light exposure. Increased dietary fat intake. There is some evidence for an inherited predisposition. Variants in the complement factor H gene, located on chromosome 1, are associated with the development of AMD.

EPIDEMIOLOGY AMD is the leading cause of blindness in the Western world amongst 50+ year-olds. Dry AMD accounts for 90% of cases of macular degeneration but can be less severe than wet AMD.

HISTORY Reduced visual acuity – gradual deterioration in central vision leading to difficulty with reading, recognizing faces, seeing fine details. Vision is not significantly improved with glasses. Metamorphopisa. Reduced contrast and colour sensitivity

EXAMINATION Drusen, focal hyperpigmentation, RPE atrophy. Geograpic atrophy can be a sign of late stage AMD. Amsler-grid testing should be used to monitor for development of wet AMD.

PATHOLOGY/PATHOGENESIS Drusen are abnormal yellow deposits located between the RPE and Bruch's membrane. These can become calcified. The overlying photoreceptors cease to function due to lack of the required support from the RPE. Geographic atrophy represents a large well demarcated area of RPE damage.

INVESTIGATIONS Optical coherence tomography, Fundus fluorescein angiography (FFA)

MANAGEMENT There is no treatment for established Dry AMD. Measures to consider to prevent progression are below.

LIFESTYLE Smoking cessation. High dose prophylcatic vitamins; C, E, zinc and beta-carotene. (Beta carotene may increase the risk of lung cancer in smokers who require a formulation without its inclusion.)

SUPPORTIVE Counselling, low vision aids, referral to support groups. Sight-impaired/severely sight-impaired registration as appropriate.

Age-related macular degeneration (AMD), dry
(continued)

COMPLICATIONS Choroidal neovascularization (wet AMD).

PROGNOSIS The presence of large drusen and pigment abnormality in one eye is associated with a 50% risk of developing AMD in the fellow eye within 5 years.

Age related macular degeneration, wet ▶

DEFINITION Degeneration of the macula complicated by choroidal neovascularization.

AETIOLOGY Unknown, likely multifactorial. Excessive secretion of vascular endothelial growth factor (VEGF) may be a cause.

ASSOCIATIONS/RISK FACTORS Increased age, female gender, smoking, hypermetropia, hypertension, alcohol intake. UV light exposure. Increased dietary fat intake. Variants in the gene coding for complement factor H, a component of the alternative complement cascade pathway, predispose to AMD.

EPIDEMIOLOGY Accounts for 10% of cases of macular degeneration, however, is responsible for most of the sight-impaired/severely sight-impaired registrations that are made in the UK.

HISTORY Subacute onset of decrease/loss of central vison +/- associated metamorphopsia.

EXAMINATION Distorted vision detectable on Amsler chart testing. Fundoscopy: subretinal fluid/haemorrhage. Macular oedema, eventual disciform scar (subretinal fibrosis).

PATHOLOGY/PATHOGENESIS There is neovascularization that develops from the choroid and extends through the RPE and into the subretinal space. The vessels are fragile and susceptible to rupture with resulting haemorrhage and oedema. Fibrosis and collagen deposition occur eventually leading to further degeneration and predisposition to bleeding of the macula. Haemorrhage and macular scarring can cause profound central vision loss.

INVESTIGATIONS Urgent fluorescein angiography – to identify choroidal neovascularization. Optical coherence topography – aids in the detection of macular oedema and has revolutionized diagnosis and monitoring of this condition.

MANAGEMENT

- *Referral to ophthalmology:* for consideration of intravitreal anti-VEGF injections.
- Amsler-grid self-monitoring (allowing patients to determine progression).

LIFESTYLE Smoking cessation/vitamin supplementation (see age-related macular degeneration, dry).

SUPPORTIVE Low-vision aids, registration as sight-impaired/severely sight-impaired, counselling, referral to support groups.

Age related macular degeneration, wet ▶
(continued)

COMPLICATIONS Without treatment permanent visual loss almost inevitable.

PROGNOSIS Intravitreal anti-VEGF injections have revolutionized treatment of wet AMD; a course of injections can lead to partial restoration of normal anatomy and cessation of the neovascularization. The benefit can be persistent.

Note: intravitreal injections can be associated with serious complications including endophthalmitis and retinal detachment.

Amaurosis fugax ▶

DEFINITION Transient monocular loss of vision.

AETIOLOGY
• There is transient interruption of the retinal blood supply. Causes of transient visual loss have been classified by the Amaurosis Fugax Study Group 1990:
• *Embolic:* cardiac/carotid
• *Haemodynamic:* arteritis, hypoperfusion, atheromatous occlusion, carotid artery dissection
• *Ocular:* anterior ischaemic optic neuropathy, retinal vessel occlusion
• *Neurological:* optic neuropathy, papilloedema, multiple sclerosis, migraine
• *Idiopathic.*

ASSOCIATIONS/RISK FACTORS Stroke, transient ischaemic attack, atherosclerosis, giant cell arteritis.

EPIDEMIOLOGY Most cases are due to underlying intracranial carotid artery disease hence the need for investigation as below to prevent stroke.

HISTORY Monocular blurring, dimming or loss of vision lasting only seconds to minutes. The classic description (which is not ubiquitous) is of a vertically descending, curtain-like loss of vision. History should include eliciting symptoms of associated pathology and risk factors in particular those of giant cell arteritis.

EXAMINATION Ophthalmic examination, especially for optic disc pallor, disc swelling and retinal ischaemia, e.g. cotton wool spots. Cholesterol emboli may be seen as small yellow deposits in the retinal arteries. A cardiac and neurological examination should be performed.

PATHOLOGY/PATHOGENESIS
• Ischaemia of the retina without infarction. The pathophysiology varies depending on the diverse underlying causes; however, the retinal circulation, with its small calibre vessels, is susceptible to obstruction by inflammation or small emboli. For example, cholesterol-rich fragments originating from atheromatous plaques in the carotid artery (Hollenhorst plaques) can temporarily obstruct the lumen of these vessels causing the symptoms.
• In other causes, the visual symptoms occur due to transient insufficiency of blood, and therefore oxygen delivery, to the retina which is highly dependent on a constant oxygen supply for its function.

Amaurosis fugax ▶ (continued)

INVESTIGATIONS For underlying pathology: BP, FBC (Increased in Polycythaemia), ESR & CRP (raised in giant cell arteritis), Fasting lipids and glucose. Carotid artery ultrasound/MRA. Cardiac echo, ECG.

MANAGEMENT

- Of the underlying cause – urgent evaluation is needed in order to initiate prompt treatment. When suspicion of giant cell arteritis is high, initiating treatment should take priority over awaiting results of investigations.
- For embolic causes, antiplatelet treatment to reduce the risk of further amaurosis fugax and stroke. Treat modifiable cardiac risk factors (hypertension, smoking, hypercholesterolaemia etc.). Carotid endarterctomy may be indicated in carotid artery disease. The Framingham equation can be used to predict a patient's 10-year cardiovascular risk.
- Patients should be advised not to drive for one month after the episode. DVLA guidance should be sought if there is recurrence of this or other neurological symptoms during this time.

COMPLICATIONS Recurrence, stroke, permanent blindness due to retinal infarction.

PROGNOSIS There is a high association with stroke. This risk is significantly reduced with carotid endarterectomy if indicated by degree of carotid artery stenosis.

Amblyopia

DEFINITION Noncorrectable poor vision due to impaired visual development.

AETIOLOGY Squint, high refractive error, anisometropia, congenital cataract, ptosis. Sensory deprivation.

ASSOCIATIONS/RISK FACTORS See above.

EPIDEMIOLOGY Prevalence of approximately 2%.

HISTORY Patients may be referred as adults with poor vision in one eye that does not improve with glasses. There may be a history of childhood squint or patching of an eye. The underlying aetiology will always be due a cause that has occurred before the age of 9 years.

EXAMINATION Poor vision in one eye that does not improve with pinhole or glasses. There may be signs of uncorrected childhood causes, as mentioned above. However, in most cases ophthalmic examination will be normal.

PATHOLOGY/PATHOGENESIS Normal development of the central nervous system's ability to process retinal images depends on focused images being presented to corresponding areas of the retina (in particular over the fovea). Poor quality images, as in the case with refractive error, or misaligned images, as in the case of squint, impair the necessary precise stimulation of the visual system. Any such interruption before the age of 9 years can lead to disruption in the development of normal visual processing and therefore permanent impairment of the vision. This process can occur bilaterally.

INVESTIGATIONS N/A.

MANAGEMENT Preventative through screening programmes for childhood detection of, for example, refractive error, squint and amblyopia. This is an important part of the work of orthoptists and school nurses. Occlusion of a better seeing eye promotes use and development of the potentially amblyopic eye. Correction of underlying causes is essential.

COMPLICATIONS Impaired vision in one eye impairs binocular stereoscopic (3D) visual perception.

PROGNOSIS Late detection or deferred treatment is associated with a worse prognosis.

Blepharitis

DEFINITION Inflammation of the eyelid margins.

AETIOLOGY Inflammation associated with one or more – excess sebum (seborrheic blepharitis) – meibomian gland dysfunction (meibomitis) – commensal bacterial overgrowth, e.g. *Staphyloccus epidermis.* Occasionally – infestation with the parasite *Demodex follicularum.*

ASSOCIATIONS/RISK FACTORS Seborrhoeic dermatitis, acne vulgaris, rosacea.

EPIDEMIOLOGY Very common. May be seen in over 40% of patients presenting to ophthalmologists.

HISTORY Chronic symptoms: grittiness, dryness or burning of the eyes. Mild intermittent visual blurring. Foreign body sensation, heavy eyelids, crusty discharge. Rarely mild photophobia.

EXAMINATION Hyperaemia of the eyelid margins and conjunctiva. Crusts and scale like deposits around the bases of the eyelashes. In severe and long-standing disease, scarring of the eyelid margin, and keratitis.

PATHOLOGY/PATHOGENESIS There is an abnormal cell-mediated inflammatory response to toxins or the cell wall components of the colonizing organisms. Excess sebum or meibomian gland oil may illicit inflammation or promote colonization with the aforementioned microorganisms.

INVESTIGATIONS Unilateral blepharitis must be investigated and treated with the presumed diagnosis of sebaceous gland carcinoma until proven otherwise.

MANAGEMENT
- *Lid hygiene and hot compresses*: round pads soaked in warm water can be used to rub the eyelids and clean the eyelid margins.
- Acute exacerbations may require topical antibiotic (such as fusidic acid) application to the eyelid margin. A short course of oral antibiotic may be indicated. Topical steroids are used to control severe associated keratitis. Dry eye should be treated with tear substitutes. An extended oral course of a tetracycline may be helpful for acute meibomian gland dysfunction.

COMPLICATIONS Dry eye, marginal keratitis, chalazion, trichiasis, conjunctivitis, ulcerative lid margin disease, entropion, ectropion.

Blepharitis (continued)

PROGNOSIS Most cases of blepharitis respond to immaculate attention to eyelid hygiene. Recurrence is common and treatment is often lifelong.

Cataract, age-related

DEFINITION An acquired opacity of the lens.

AETIOLOGY Increased age, cumulative damage from sun exposure.

ASSOCIATIONS/RISK FACTORS Smoking. Systemic disease, e.g. DM. Ocular diseases, e.g. uveitis, infection. Drugs, e.g. corticiosteroids. Inborn or acquired errors of metabolism, trauma, radiation.

EPIDEMIOLOGY Causes 50% of worldwide blindness.

HISTORY Painless decline of vision, blurred vision, glare, diplopia (monocular), change in refractive error.

EXAMINATION On direct ophthalmoscopy there may be loss of the red reflex or, more commonly, cataracts may appear as dark opacities against the red reflex.

PATHOLOGY Dysregulation of lens metabolism secondary to the reduced efficiency of antioxidant defence mechanisms, such as those involving glutathione. Disordered packing of the lens crystallin proteins causing disruption of light transmission. Increased light scatter (which manifests as glare) caused by an increased water content in the lens.

INVESTIGATIONS
- Diagnosis is normally made clinically on slit lamp. If cataract precludes adequate funduscopy then posterior segment ultrasound is indicated.
- *Biometry:* to measure the curvature of the cornea (keratometry) and axial length (e.g. A-scan ultrasound) in order to calculate the required intraocular lens implant power.

MANAGEMENT

INDICATIONS FOR SURGERY A decline in vision that affects activities of daily living. Restoration of clarity of optical media in order to permit visualization for monitoring and treatment of retinal pathology, e.g. diabetic retinopathy. For cosmetic purposes; such as for the removal of a cataract in an eye blinded by another cause.

SURGERY Phacoemulsification (procedure of choice in the developed world). This involves liquification of the cataract using an ultrasound probe through a small, self-healing incision and implantation of an intraocular lens.

Cataract, age-related (continued)

COMPLICATIONS OF SURGERY Macular oedema, posterior capsular •
opacification (clouding of the capsular membrane that is left in-situ),
inflammation (iritis) and unexpected refractive error. Rarely
endophthalmitis and intraocular bleeding (may cause permanent visual
loss; rare).

PROGNOSIS Continued slow loss of vision without surgery.

Cataract, congenital

DEFINITION Opacity of the lens present at, or shortly after, birth.

AETIOLOGY Intrauterine infections: TORCH infections (toxoplamosis, other, rubella, cytomegalovirus, herpes). 'Other' includes coxsackievirus, HIV, syphilis and Varicella-Zoster virus. Inborn errors of metabolism; e.g. galactosaemia, chromosome defects; trisomy, Turner's syndrome. Myotonic Dystrophy. Idiopathic.

ASSOCIATIONS/RISK FACTORS Family history. Metabolic or systemic disease is found in 60% of cases. See above.

EPIDEMIOLOGY Incidence 1/10 000.

HISTORY Parents may note a white pupil or squint in their child. Most will be detected at routine health checks. Some may not present until adulthood despite the cataract having been present since birth.

EXAMINATION Leukocoria. Abnormal red reflex. Squint or nystagmus may be present. Gross visual function can be assessed by observing the child's ability to fix on and follow targets. Orthoptist assessment is indicated. Dysmorphic features suggestive of chromosomal abnormalities may be noted.

PATHOLOGY/PATHOGENESIS Any insult to the developing lens fibres during gestation can lead to lens opacity hence the wide ranging aetiology.

INVESTIGATIONS Serology (TORCH), fasting blood glucose. Specialist tests for metabolic diseases and chromosomal abnormalities are best directed by paediatricians/paediatric ophthalmologists.

MANAGEMENT There should be prompt referral to paediatric ophthalmology. Retinoblastoma is an important and potentially fatal differential diagnosis for leukocoria. Treatment is aimed and preventing amblyopia. Early surgery for bilateral congenital cataract is advocated whilst surgery for unilateral disease is more controversial.

COMPLICATIONS Amblyopia, glaucoma, retinal detachment.

PROGNOSIS There is significant risk of amblyopia without proper postoperative visual rehabilitation and close long-term follow-up is required

Cavernous sinus syndrome ▶

DEFINITION A syndrome caused by a lesion that give rise to a mass effect within the cavernous sinus.

AETIOLOGY Cavernous sinus tumours (primary or metastatic), cavernous sinus thrombosis (may be due to infection with *Staphylococcus aureus or Streptococcus pneumoniae*), cavernous sinus aneurysm, carotid-cavernous fistula. Inflammatory causes – Tolosa Hunt syndrome. Sarcoidosis.

ASSOCIATIONS/RISK FACTORS Increased age – cavernous sinus aneurysms, trauma; can cause carotid-cavernous sinus fistulas. Sarcoidosis. Wegener granulomatosis. Facial infection.

EPIDEMIOLOGY Uncommon.

HISTORY Reduced vision, protrusion of the eye, red eye, diplopia, painful eye movements, headache. Concurrent infection of the face, sinuses or dentition. Symptoms are usually unilateral but may be bilateral.

EXAMINATION
May be systemically unwell (e.g. fever, tachycardia).

Multiple cranial nerve palsies
- II – reduced vision, RAPD and decreased colour perception – if there is primary orbital involvement.
- III, IV, VI - painful ophthalmolplegia and ptosis.
- V_{1-2} (ophthalmic and maxillary divisions) reduced/absent sensation including corneal reflex.

Specific additional signs
- Pulsating exophthalmos, conjunctival/lid oedema – direct carotid-cavernous-fistula.
- Visual field defect, endocrinological signs – pituitary tumours.
- Local and systemic signs of infection, meningism, papilloedema – cavernous sinus thrombosis.

PATHOLOGY/PATHOGENESIS The cavernous sinuses are paired intracranial venous structures bounded by the sphenoid bone and temporal bone that communicate with the ophthalmic veins. Traversing through the cavity are important structures including the internal carotid artery, CNIII, CNIV, CNV_{1-2}, CNVI. Mass effect or thrombosis within the cavity therefore leads to the signs described above. Tolosa Hunt syndrome is an ideopathic inflammation of the walls of the cavernous sinus. The pituitary gland lies medial to the cavernous sinus thus pituitary tumour or apoplexy can impinge on the structures within it.

Cavernous sinus syndrome ▶ (continued)

INVESTIGATIONS Urgent neuroimaging: MRI/MRA/MRV. CT of the orbit/nasal sinuses. FBC, blood cultures, ESR. Lumbar puncture for cytological analysis.

MANAGEMENT
- Urgent referral to the appropriate speciality.
- Tumours – radiotherapy, resection.
- Cavernous sinus thrombosis – antibiotics, drainage of site of primary infection.
- Inflammatory causes (e.g. Tolosa hunt syndrome) – systemic steroids.
- Cavernous sinus aneurysms, carotid-cavernous fistulas – endovascular neurosurgical intervention.

COMPLICATIONS Death, meningitis, sepsis, cerebral abscess, blindness, permanent cranial nerve palsy.

PROGNOSIS Fatal in 20–30% of cases.

Cellulitis, orbital ▶

DEFINITION Soft tissue infection of orbital tissue (posterior to the orbital septum).

AETIOLOGY Common pathogens include *Staphylococcus aureus, Streptococcus pneumoniae, Staphylococcus epidermidis, Streptococcus pyogenes.*

ASSOCIATIONS/RISK FACTORS Preseptal cellulitis (especially in children). Penetrating eyelid trauma, sinusitis.

EPIDEMIOLOGY Rare. Most occur in association with sinusitis.

HISTORY Fever, anorexia, malaise, eyelid and periocular pain, with swelling. Double/blurred vision. Painful eye movements. Commonly there are preceding upper respiratory tract/sinusitis symptoms.

EXAMINATION Pyrexia. Periorbital erythema/oedema/tenderness. Restricted and painful eye movements. Proptosis. Reduced visual acuity, RAPD.

PATHOLOGY/PATHOGENESIS The orbital septum in children is under-developed and provides less of a barrier to infection than in adults hence the importance of close monitoring in children with pre-septal cellulitis. Infection can spread from other adjacent sites of infection (e.g. dental abscess/dacrocystitis).

INVESTIGATIONS FBC, blood cultures, CT – orbits/brain/sinus.

MANAGEMENT Admit – urgent referral to paediatrics (in children) with ophthalmology and ENT involvement. IV antibiotics, e.g. flucloxacillin. Regular monitoring of observations and of optic nerve function. Surgical drainage in nonresponsive cases.

COMPLICATIONS Orbital cellulitis is a sight threatening and potentially fatal condition. A compressive optic neuropathy can occur and rarely cavernous sinus syndrome, meningitis or intracranial abscess formation can occur.

PROGNOSIS Good if recognized and treated promptly.

Cellulitis, preseptal

DEFINITION Infection limited to subcutaneous tissue anterior to the orbital septum.

AETIOLOGY *Staphylococcus aureus* and *Streptococcal Sp.* are common causative organisms arising from adjacent sites, contamination is usually from traumatic skin puncture or haematogenous spread.

ASSOCIATIONS/RISK FACTORS Upper respiratory tract infection, cuts to the eyelid skin, insect bites, infected chalazia, dacrocystitis, dental infection.

EPIDEMIOLOGY Common, especially in children.

HISTORY Eyelid swelling and tenderness.

EXAMINATION Erythema of eyelids with oedema and tenderness. Typically a white eye with normal visual acuity, colour vision, pupil reflexes and eye movements. Usually unilateral. No systemic upset/pyrexia.

PATHOLOGY/PATHOGENESIS The causative organisms reflect those found as commensals on the eyelids or upper respiratory tract. There is no penetration of infection through to the orbital septum. The orbital septum separates the subcutaneous eyelid tissue from the deeper orbital structures and provides a barrier to infection. This may not be fully developed in children hence their increased risk of developing orbital cellulitis and systemic complications.

INVESTIGATIONS To exclude orbital cellulites (see **p. 51**).

MANAGEMENT Oral antibiotics, e.g. flucloxacillin. Regular review until resolution. Children require admission with paediatric/ophthalmology/ENT review. ▶

COMPLICATIONS Orbital cellulitis.

PROGNOSIS Good with prompt recognition and treatment.

Chemical injury to the eye ▶

DEFINITION Accidental or intentional exposure of the eye to chemical agents with potentially blinding complications.

AETIOLOGY Assault, accidental.

ASSOCIATIONS/RISK FACTORS Industrial chemical exposure.

EPIDEMIOLOGY Common source of eye injuries presenting to A&E.

HISTORY Most patients will remember a chemical insult. They will complain of pain, photophobia, reduced vision, and difficulty in eye opening. It is essential to ascertain the chemical agent if possible.

EXAMINATION
- Should be preceded by urgent irrigation as below and measurement of pH if available. This is assuming that there are not more pressing life-threatening injuries needing attention.
- The eye will typically be red; however severe injury can lead to the appearance of a white conjunctiva as all of the vessels are blanched. The cornea will be opacified in severe injuries. Whiteness of the limbus can suggest limbal ischaemia.
- Slit lamp examination may show anterior chamber inflammation.
- The chemical agent may cause facial burns or burns elsewhere which must be appropriately assessed and treated. Ophthalmologists will monitor intraocular pressures if they are concerned about inflammation in the anterior chamber.

PATHOLOGY/PATHOGENESIS
- Alkali injuries are frequently more severe than those caused by acids. Due to saponification of fatty acids in cell membranes, alkali can penetrate deep into the eye and lead to substantial intraocular inflammation and damage.
- Damage from strong acids can be no less severe; however, in most cases, acids will lead to the denaturing of proteins on the surface of the eye, thus creating a barrier to further penetration of the chemical agent.
- The limbal stem cells are responsible for maintaining the corneal epithelium hence the concern from limbal ischaemia.

INVESTIGATIONS pH measurement.

Chemical injury to the eye ▶ (continued)

MANAGEMENT
- Immediate irrigation of the eye with normal saline.
- Eye opening may be maintained with an eyelid speculum and a drop of topical anaesthetic after pH measurement. Irrigation should continue until the pH is 7.0–7.5. Swabs should be used to sweep away any particulate matter including that which may have accumulated under the eyelids.
- Mild injury with a clear cornea and no limbal ischaemia may not need ophthalmology follow-up.
- More severe injury may require treatment to control raised intraocular pressures, inflammation or promote healing of the corneal epithelium. Severe injury may need treatment with amniotic membrane grafting, limbal stem cell transplant or corneal transplant.

COMPLICATIONS Glaucoma, cataract, permanent corneal opacification.

PROGNOSIS Corneal opacification (iris details obscured) and limbal ischaemia are adverse prognostic factors.

Conjunctivitis, bacterial and chlamydial

DEFINITION Infection of the conjunctiva.

AETIOLOGY Common organisms include *Staphylococcus epidermidis*, *Staphylococcus aureus* and *Haemophilus influenzea*. The latter occurs most commonly in children. Propionibacterium acnes, *Moraxella catarrhalis* and Corneybacterium can also become pathogens. *Neisseria gonorrhoeae* is a rare but serious cause of conjunctivitis, especially in neonates (*Ophthalmia neonatorum* – see below). *Chlamydia trachomatis* is an important cause of conjunctivitis that in the UK is most often a sexually transmitted infection. Spread can occur with direct contact.

ASSOCIATIONS/RISK FACTORS Contact with infected people. Eyelid disorders such as entropion and trichiasis. Immunocompromised patients are predisposed to atypical pathogens.

EPIDEMIOLOGY Very common.

HISTORY Acute onset of a sticky red eye. Patients may complain of grittiness. One eye may be affected initially but bilateral infection commonly follows. *Chlamydia trachomatis* is often unilateral and can have a subacute onset with a prolonged course.

EXAMINATION Normal visual acuity (or may be slightly and transiently reduced due to discharge).Red eye (conjunctival injection), conjunctival chemosis, mucopurulent discharge, crusting of the eyelids. *Neisserria gonorrhoea* induces a particularly purulent discharge and may cause a keratitis.

PATHOLOGY/PATHOGENESIS
- The eyelids, tears and conjunctiva all contribute to the eye's defence against microbial infection. Bacteria must overcome these to cause infection. For example, *Neisserria gonorrhoea* can penetrate an intact conjunctival and corneal epithelium. Invasion by other organisms can be mediated by abrasion of the epithelium (for example in the presence of trichiasis) or by bacterial toxin and enzyme production (for example with *Staphylococcus aureus* infection).
- The infected conjunctival epithelium becomes oedematous and there is a polymorphonuclear leukocyte inflammatory infiltrate.

INVESTIGATIONS None in almost all cases. Severe and recurrent infections, or those occurring in neonates and the immunosuppressed, should prompt culture and sensitivity testing of conjunctival swabs. Chronic cases should also warrant investigation.

Conjunctivitis, bacterial and chlamydial (continued)

MANAGEMENT Almost all cases can be managed in primary care. Topical ophthalmic preparations of chloramphenicol (or fuscidic acid) are often effective in bacterial conjunctivitis. Ointments smear vision but will require less frequent administration than drop (guttae) preparations. *Neisseria* and *chlamydial* conjunctivitis in the adult is a sexually transmitted infection that requires systemic antibiotics and referral to a genitourinary clinic. Paediatric neisseria and chlamydia infections require urgent hospital admission and treatment.

Hygiene advice: Hand washing, no sharing of towels, no touching the eyes.

COMPLICATIONS
- Otitis can develop in children with *Haemophilus influenzae* infection. *Staphyloccus aureus* infection can lead to chronic conjunctivitis and blepharitis. *Neisseria gonorrhoea* can penetrate the cornea and lead to its ulceration and subsequent perforation.
- *Chlamydia trachomatis,* serotypes Ab, B, Ba, or C, can cause trachoma which accounts for most of the preventable blindness in the world. Trachoma occurs due to progressive conjunctival scarring which leads to trichiasis, entropion and subsequent visually devastating corneal scarring.

PROGNOSIS Most cases of simple bacterial conjunctivitis will resolve spontaneously within a week. Antimicrobial treatment can quicken recovery.

Conjunctivitis, other (including ophthalmia neonatorum) ▶

Allergic conjunctivitis

Bilateral itchy eyes with watering, especially in atopic individuals or those with allergies. Signs include red eyes with chemosis and conjunctival papillae. Underlying causes should be eliminated if possible. Topical lubricants, over the counter anti-allergy drops, or oral antihistamines may help.

Ophthalmia neonatorum ▶

- This is microbial conjunctivitis occurring in the first month of life. Chlamydia is associated with profuse mucopurulent discharge. *Neisseria gonorrhoea* causes a severe conjunctivitis (see above) and can be associated with meningitis. Urgent treatment is needed for *Ophthalmia neonatorum* to prevent potential visual loss and morbidity and death!
- Swabs for microscopy, culture and sensitivity should be taken and systemic antimicrobial treatment started. For example, erythromycin for chlamydial and ceftriaxone for gonococcal causes. The mother should also be investigated and treated if needed.

Conjunctivitis, viral

DEFINITION Viral Infection of the conjunctiva.

AETIOLOGY Viral conjunctivitis is very easily spread through direct contact with ocular secretions, aerosol of respiratory secretions or fomite contact. Viruses can survive for hours on surfaces, such as examination instruments and magazines in patient waiting rooms. The most common infective agent is adenovirus. Molluscum contagiosum and herpes simplex infection can also give rise to conjunctivitis. These examples are all dsDNA viruses.

ASSOCIATIONS/RISK FACTORS Contact with infected individuals. Molluscum contagiosum and herpes simplex can lead to profuse reactions in Aids sufferers or the immunocompomised.

EPIDEMIOLOGY Overall incidence <1%. However, viral conjunctivitis can occur in epidemics that are sometimes traced back to ophthalmology clinics! Adenovirus is typically implicated; often in conjunction with an upper respiratory tract infection (pharyngoconjunctivitis).

HISTORY Acute onset, red, watery eye with burning/grittiness. If bilateral, history may reveal a unilateral onset. Associated keratitis can occur with photophobia and blurred vision.

EXAMINATION
- Watering, red eye, conjunctival chemosis, follicles (on eversion of the eyelid). Eyelid oedema may occur as may conjunctival haemorrhage and pseudo-membrane formation. Vision is most often normal. If there is blurring, this may be due to excessive watering or corneal involvement.
- Tender palpable pre-auricular lymphadenopathy in adenoviral infection.
- Slit lamp examination: keratoconjunctivitis – corneal involvement (fine fluorescein staining with or without diffuse fine opacities).
- Molluscum contagiosum: pearly surfaced, umbilicated, nodule(s) near the eyelid may be apparent.
- Herpes simplex: vesicles may be apparent on the eyelid. Dendritic ulcers may be seen on the cornea with slit lamp examination and fluorescein staining (see 'Keratitis, herpetic', **p. 91**).

Conjunctivitis, viral (continued)
PATHOLOGY/PATHOGENESIS
- Adenovirus is a dsDNA virus with a multitude of serotypes. It has an incubation period of 7 days. There is a long period over which communicability is high as active virus particles continue to be shed for two weeks following onset of symptoms.
- The mildest cases of viral conjunctivitis have no systemic or corneal involvement (simple follicular conjunctivitis).
- Molluscum contagiosum – infection of the eyelid causes conjunctivitis as viral particles are shed onto the conjunctiva.
- Herpes simplex – active herpes simplex disease can be a sign of primary infection or reactivation of the virus which can reside dormant in cranial nerve ganglia.

INVESTIGATIONS Viral PCR of conjunctival swabs – rarely performed.

MANAGEMENT
- Simple follicular conjunctivitis – supportive; cold compresses over the eyelids or artificial tears may provide some symptomatic relief. Strict hygiene must be emphasized, e.g. hand washing, avoiding close contact, not sharing towels.
- The nodular lesions of molluscum contagiosum can be excised.
- Herpes simplex infection may warrant topical aciclovir.

COMPLICATIONS Chronic adenoviral keratoconjunctivitis – recurrent exacerbations of symptoms with corneal involvement (see below).

PROGNOSIS Virtually all resolve with no consequence, although symptoms may persist for several weeks.

NOTE ON ADENOVIRAL KERATITIS Severe keratitis can complicate adenoviral conjunctivitis caused by serotypes 8, 19 and 37. The cornea may initially demonstrate a diffuse punctate staining pattern followed by the development of sub-epithelial deposits. Treatment is supportive. Topical steroids are occasionally used, and with great caution, once active lesions become quiescent.

Cranial nerve III (CNIII) palsy ▶

DEFINITION Lesion of the third cranial nerve (occulomotor nerve).

AETIOLOGY
- Ischaemic vascular disease: most common and usually secondary to diabetes or hypertension
- Vasculitis
- Intracranial compressive lesions (aneurysm, haematoma secondary to trauma, malignancy, pituitary apoplexy)
- Demyelination

ASSOCIATIONS/RISK FACTORS Poorly controlled hypertension/ diabetes, head injury.

EPIDEMIOLOGY
Uncommon. Incidence <1% of diabetics. One-third patients with a posterior communicating artery aneurysm have a CNIII palsy.

HISTORY
- Droopy eyelid, double vision. Patients will often present with a droopy eyelid and not complain of diplopia because the affected eye will is covered. As the ptosis resolves the diplopia may become apparent to a patient.
- History should rule out potentially fatal pathology so ask about trauma and symptoms of raised intracranial pressure (sudden onset severe headache, vomiting, loss of consciousness).

EXAMINATION Ptosis. The affected eye will be directed 'down and out' (depressed and abducted). The pupil may or may not be dilated and nonreactive (see below). Diplopia in primary gaze may be elicited on elevation of the closed eyelid.

PATHOLOGY/PATHOGENESIS

DIPLOPIA Secondary to unopposed action of the lateral rectus and superior oblique (the only two ocular muscles not supplied by CNIII).

PTOSIS Due to loss of supply to the levator palpebrae superioris.

PUPIL SIGNS The blood supply to the CNIII is formed of two components. The pial vessels supply the superficial fibres of the nerve where the parasympathetic pupillary fibres traverse. Typically diabetic or hypertensive microvascular disease only affects the blood supply to the central part of the third nerve which carries fibres to the ocular muscles. Microvascular disease can therefore affect the third nerve but not give rise to a dilated pupil – (a medical CNIII palsy or 'partial, pupil sparing' CNIII palsy). An extrinsic compressive lesion would unselectively affect the CNIII and thus cause a 'complete' or 'surgical' CNIII palsy with pupil and motor signs.

Cranial nerve III (CNIII) palsy ▶ (continued)

WARNING The above signs are not rules that are always obeyed and evolve over time so cannot be relied upon to rule out a potentially fatal intracranial lesion.

INVESTIGATIONS Consider urgent MRA. BP, blood glucose, ESR, fasting lipids.

MANAGEMENT

MEDICAL Management of diabetes, hypertension and other vascular risk factors. Otherwise depends on the underlying cause. Diplopia may require patching of the affected eye or the prescription of glasses with prisms.

SURGICAL Urgent neurosurgical intervention if an intracranial lesion is present.

COMPLICATIONS Death if an intracranial compressive lesion remains undiagnosed/untreated. Persistent diplopia.

PROGNOSIS Most will resolve independent of the cause if underlying pathology is managed. Persistent diplopia or ptosis may warrant surgery.

Cranial nerve IV (CNIV) palsy ▶

DEFINITION Palsy of CNIV, the trochlear nerve.

AETIOLOGY Congenital (although may not present until adulthood). Head injury. Microvascular disease secondary to diabetes, hypertension, or atherosclerosis. Rarely; aneurysms, tumours, vasculitis.

ASSOCIATIONS/RISK FACTORS Most cases are idiopathic and head trauma accounts for most other causes.

EPIDEMIOLOGY Rare.

HISTORY Vertical diplopia, Squint, head tilt (may be noticed from photographs in congenital cases). Sudden/recent onset symptoms associated with head trauma.

EXAMINATION Ipsilateral hypertropia (manifest vertical squint), limited depression of the affected eye. Diplopia worse on downgaze. Contralateral head tilt.

PATHOLOGY/PATHOGENESIS CNIV is a long nerve that arises from the dorsal aspect of the brain. The trunk of the nerve passes over the rigid edge of the tentorium. It is therefore susceptible to minor head trauma causing 'stretch' of the nerve. Bilateral CNIV palsy occurs in cases of such intracranial pathology. CNIV supplies the superior oblique which is responsible for depression (when the eye is adducted) and intorsion of the eye (when the eye is abducted) explaining the compensatory head tilt.

INVESTIGATIONS Consider neuroimaging in acute cases. BP, FBC, ESR, lipids, glucose.

MANAGEMENT Treat the underlying cause. Patching/prisms. Squint surgery.

COMPLICATIONS Persistent diplopia.

PROGNOSIS Medical causes have a high rate of spontaneous recovery. Definitive surgical management is often needed in traumatic causes due to low rates of spontaneous recovery.

Cranial nerve VI (CNVI) palsy ▶

DEFINITION Palsy of CNVI, the abducens nerve.

AETIOLOGY Microvascular disease secondary to diabetes or hypertension, basal skull fractures, raised intracranial pressure, demyelination, vasculitis, tumours.

ASSOCIATIONS/RISK FACTORS May be associated with raised intracranial pressure (a false localizing sign; see below). Pontine gliomas in children can give rise to this lesion. Posterior fossa tumour resection.

EPIDEMIOLOGY CNVI is the most commonly affected ocular motor nerve.

HISTORY Double vision on the horizontal plane, worse on looking in the direction of the affected muscle. Squint. Symptoms of raised intracranial pressure should be excluded.

EXAMINATION Esotropia (manifest convergent squint) of the affected eye; worse when looking into the distance than near. Limited abduction. Head turn, towards the affected side. Cranial nerve examination should be performed with particular attention to hearing and the corneal reflex

PATHOLOGY/PATHOGENESIS
- CNVI supplies the lateral rectus hence the esotropia and limited abduction. The head turns towards the affected side to reduce the consequential diplopia.
- The nerve is prone to stretching over the petrous tip in cases of raised intracranial pressure or tumours which can cause the brainstem to become displaced inferiorly. This can give rise to a falsely localizing sign in that a patient may appear to have an isolated CNVI palsy but actually have life-threatening intracranial pathology.
- Pontine gliomas can present with this sign. Acoustic neuromas may damage the 6th nerve although CNVI palsy alone will rarely be a presenting feature.

INVESTIGATIONS BP, FBC, glucose, lipids, ESR. Low threshold for neuroimaging in the young or if there is no resolution within three months in adults. Multiple cranial nerve signs should prompt urgent MRI.

MANAGEMENT Depending on underlying cause. Persistent symptoms despite treatment of the underlying cause may require prisms to be incorporated into a glasses prescription, eye patching or squint surgery.

Cranial nerve VI (CNVI) palsy ▶ (continued)

COMPLICATIONS Persistence of diplopia. Some underlying causes have fatal sequelae if not identified and managed.

PROGNOSIS Spontaneous recovery is common in those with an underlying microvascular cause.

Cytomegalovirus (CMV) retinitis ▶

DEFINITION Inflammation of the retina caused by cytomegalovirus.

AETIOLOGY Reactivation or opportunistic infection by CMV.

ASSOCIATIONS/RISK FACTORS AIDS (CD4+ count - <50 cells/ml), immunosuppression.

EPIDEMIOLOGY The most common ocular infection in AIDS; rare otherwise. The prevalence of previous (typically asymptomatic) systemic infection with CMV in the general population is >50%.

HISTORY Blurred vision, visual field defect. Photophobia or eye pain may be features.

EXAMINATION Patchy white areas of retina (necrosis), retinal haemorrhage (pizza-pie, bush-fire appearance). Other signs such as inflammation in the vitreous may be detected by an ophthalmologist examining with a slit lamp.

PATHOLOGY/PATHOGENESIS CMV is a DNA virus. It causes the appearance of intranuclear inclusion bodies in infected cells. Intraretinal proliferation leads to inflammation and necrosis of the retina.

INVESTIGATIONS HIV test (if undiagnosed), CD4 count.

MANAGEMENT By an ophthalmologist and HIV physician. May require systemic or intravitreal ganciclovir and HAART (highly active antiretroviral treatment). Some centres employ screening of HIV patients with CD4+ counts of <50 cells/ml.

COMPLICATIONS Retinal detachment, optic nerve involvement.

PROGNOSIS Most cases respond to treatment. Untreated bilateral disease is frequent. Recurrence is common.

Dacrocystitis ▶

DEFINITION Infection of the lacrimal sac.

AETIOLOGY Staphylococcal or streptococcal infection most common.

ASSOCIATIONS/RISK FACTORS Normal anatomic variants: narrow face/flat nose. Brachycephaly.

EPIDEMIOLOGY Occurs more often in infants and adults over 40 years. Rare in Black race.

HISTORY Varying degrees of pain, subacute onset, at the site of an erythematous swelling. Epiphora.

EXAMINATION Tender swelling below the medial canthus. Preseptal cellulitis may be present. Pyrexia if severe.

PATHOLOGY/PATHOGENESIS Nasolacrimal duct obstruction prevents normal drainage from the lacrimal sac and leads to tear retention. Infection occurs secondary to chronic tear stasis.

INVESTIGATIONS Nil; consider swab for M,C &S.

MANAGEMENT Warm compresses. Oral antibiotics. Consider incision and drainage. Severe cases, or when orbital cellulitis is present, warrant parenteral antibiotics. Dacrocystorhinostomy should be considered following subsidence of the acute infection to prevent recurrence.

COMPLICATIONS Orbital cellulitis. Mucocoele formation in the lacrimal sac. Chronic dacrocyctitis.

PROGNOSIS Recurrence is common and subacute infection can persist until successful surgical intervention.

Diabetic retinopathy

DEFINITION A microvascular complication of diabetes mellitus (DM).

AETIOLOGY Diabetes mellitus causes damage to the microvascular supply of the retina.

ASSOCIATIONS/RISK FACTORS Long duration since onset of diabetes, uncontrolled hypertension, poor diabetic control, hypercholesterolaemia. Nephropathy and pregnancy can accelerate progression of diabetic retinopathy.

EPIDEMIOLOGY Rarely a feature on presentation of Type 1 diabetics but will affect 90% within 15 years. Can be a feature on presentation of Type 2 diabetics due to common delays between onset of diabetes and its identification/control. Will affect >50% within 15 years.

HISTORY Asymptomatic in initial stages. Ask about diabetic/hypertension control. Advanced disease: blurred vision, distortion, floaters.

EXAMINATION

Nonproliferative
- Microaneurysms – small red dots in the retina.
- Blot haemorrhages – localized red haemorrhages within the retina.
- Flame-shaped haemorrhages – superficial haemorrhages in the retinal nerve fibre layer.
- Hard exudates – retinal yellow lesions with distinct margins.
- Cotton wool spots – indistinct superficial pale/white retinal lesions.
- Venous loops and venous beading – sausage shaped retinal venules.
- Macular oedema – retinal thickening that requires slit lamp microscopy or ocular coherence tomography to be appreciated.

Proliferative
- New retinal blood vessels.

Classification (simplified)
- *Nonproliferative* diabetic retinopathy – graded as mild, moderate or severe depending upon the number and severity of the above signs.
- *Diabetic maculopathy* – macular oedema and hard exudates close to the fovea are the most common cause of visual symptoms in diabetic retinopathy.
- *Proliferative diabetic retinopathy* – characterized by neovascularization at the disc (NVD) or elsewhere (NVE).

Diabetic retinopathy (continued)

PATHOLOGY/PATHOGENESIS Hyperglycaemia mediates damage to the pericytes of capillary walls. Weakened walls are prone to out-pouching (microaneurysms). These microaneurysms (dots) are prone to rupture (causing blot or flame haemorrhages). Damage to capillary endothelium predisposes to plasma leakage. Resultant collections of lipids, proteins and macrophages manifest as hard exudates. Capillary closure induces ischaemia. In the retina, nerve fibre infarction and subsequent swelling causes cotton wool spots. Other features of ischaemia are widespread haemorrhages and venous beading. New vessel growth is stimulated by VEGF (vascular endothelial growth factor) production by the ischaemic retina.

INVESTIGATIONS Blood pressure. Blood glucose, HbA1c. Lipid profile. Urine dipstick. Fundus fluorescein angiography allowing imaging and accurate diagnosis of the stage of retinopathy/detection of vessel leakage/retinal ischaemia.

MANAGEMENT
- The most important management aspect is good diabetic control, including control of risk factors. Smoking cessation, exercise and weight control are also beneficial.
- Management of retinopathy is usually coordinated between diabetic retinopathy screening services and ophthalmologists. Mild nonproliferative diabetic retinopathy can be monitored annually. More severe retinopathy may require laser photocoagulation. Increasingly anti-VEGF agents are being used in such cases.

COMPLICATIONS Iris neovascularization and secondary glaucoma. Vitreous haemorrhage. Retinal detachment. Blindness.

PROGNOSIS 5% will become blind.

Ectropion

DEFINITION Outward turning of the eyelid.

AETIOLOGY Congenital, neurological, involutional (age-related), cicatricial.

ASSOCIATIONS/RISK FACTORS Increased age, UV mediated skin damage, chemical/thermal eyelid injury.

EPIDEMIOLOGY Prevalence of 20% in those aged over 80 years.

HISTORY Dry eye, epiphora, out-turned eyelid appearance.

EXAMINATION The eyelid margin is turned away from the surface of the eye. Conjunctival injection. The cornea may show signs of drying. Neurological causes may show facial nerve palsy with lagophthalmos. Scarring will be apparent in cicatrical causes.

PATHOLOGY/PATHOGENESIS
* Facial nerve palsy is the most common neurological cause of ectropion and lagophthalmos.
* Age is associated with excessive laxity of the supporting structures of the eyelid, including the medial and lateral canthal tendons. Overriding layers of orbicularis oculi muscle are also implicated.

INVESTIGATIONS None.

MANAGEMENT
* *Symptomatic:* tear substitutes.
* *Definitive:* surgical correction.

COMPLICATIONS Exposure keratopathy. The conjunctival surface of the lower eyelid can become keratinized and inflamed.

PROGNOSIS Surgical treatment is often effective.

Endophthalmitis ▶

DEFINITION Sight threatening intraocular infection.

AETIOLOGY Most cases are exogenous; postoperative or traumatic, occurring due to inoculation of bacteria into the eye. Following surgery, the source is often the eyelid flora and infective organisms include *Staphyloccus epidermidis, Staphyloccus aureus, Streptococci pneumoniae, Haemophilus influenzae.* Endogenous endophthalmitis can also occur, e.g. following candidaemia.

ASSOCIATIONS/RISK FACTORS Postoperatively; age, complicated surgery, poor aseptic technique. Trauma; delayed primary wound closure and type of penetrating injury.

EPIDEMIOLOGY Occurs as a complication affecting approximately 0.1% of small incision cataract procedures.

HISTORY Acute presentation soon after intraocular surgery (later in low-grade chronic cases). Severe pain, deterioration of vision, worsening of redness, epiphora, photophobia.

EXAMINATION Reduced vision. Inflamed and red eye. Swollen eyelids. Relative afferent pupillary defect, abnormal red reflex, corneal haze. Hypopyon. The fundus may not be visible with an ophthalmoscope.

PATHOLOGY/PATHOGENESIS Bacterial toxins and intraocular inflammation cause direct and permanent photoreceptor damage.

INVESTIGATIONS B-Scan ultrasound if no fundal view. Anterior chamber fluid and vitreous samples are obtained for microbial investigation.

MANAGEMENT Urgent referral to an ophthalmologist – management will include obtaining diagnostic specimens as above and instillation of intravitreal antibiotics in theatre. Systemic antibiotic and steroid administration, as well and their topical instillation, are indicated.

COMPLICATIONS Persistent inflammation. Severe infection requiring enucleation or evisceration. Sympathetic ophthalmia – a bilateral granulomatous uveitis that is very rare and occurs after surgery or trauma to one eye.

PROGNOSIS Poor if the infection is severe or inadequately treated.

Entropion

DEFINITION Inward turning of the eyelid.

AETIOLOGY Involutional (age-related), congenital, cicatricial.

ASSOCIATIONS/RISK FACTORS Increased age.

EPIDEMIOLOGY More common in females than males.

HISTORY Patients may complain of eyelashes irritating the eye and/or a foreign body sensation with watering.

EXAMINATION The lower eyelid is usually affected. Eyelashes may be seen rubbing against the ocular surface. The eyelid margin will be turned towards the ocular surface. The corneal surface should be examined for erosions. The conjunctiva may be injected.

PATHOLOGY/PATHOGENESIS
- Age-related degeneration of the eyelid's supporting structures causes eyelid laxity.
- Cicatricial – conjunctival injury predisposes to scar formation and posterior eyelid shortening causing in turning. Trachoma is a common cause of upper eyelid entropion.

INVESTIGATIONS None.

MANAGEMENT Surgical entropion repair with eyelid tightening is the definitive management. Botulinium toxin injection can be used as a temporary treatment.

COMPLICATIONS Corneal ulceration.

PROGNOSIS Good following surgery.

Episcleritis

DEFINITION Mild inflammation of the episclera.

AETIOLOGY Most cases are idiopathic.

ASSOCIATIONS/RISK FACTORS Connective tissue disorders, vasculitis, gout, sarcoidosis. Infectious – tuberculosis, syphillis, herpes zoster.

EPIDEMIOLOGY Increased prevalence amongst females.

HISTORY Rapid onset (often within hours) ache/discomfort of the eye – mild. Worse on eye movements.

EXAMINATION Normal vision. There may be diffuse or sectoral vasodilation of radially orientated episcleral vessels. There may be a nodule underlying inflamed vessels. There may be mild tenderness localized to the area of inflammation. There will be no intraocular inflammation. Instillation of 10% phenylephrine will blanch these vessels assisting in the distinction between episcleritis and scleritis.

PATHOLOGY/PATHOGENESIS The superficial episcleral plexus lies between the conjunctival layer and sclera. Typically there is a local nongranulomatous inflammation affecting this vascular network (granulomatous in TB or sarcoid).

INVESTIGATIONS None needed unless underlying infectious/autoimmune/systemic disease suspected.

MANAGEMENT Often no treatment is needed. Lubricant eye drops can treat any overlying conjunctival tear disturbance. Topical steroids or systemic NSAIDs such as flurbiprofen are effective in refractory cases.

COMPLICATIONS None. Recurrence is not infrequent.

PROGNOSIS There is a good prognosis.

Exposure keratopathy

DEFINITION Corneal damage secondary inadequate ocular surface protection.

AETIOLOGY Lagophthalmos (incomplete eye closure).

ASSOCIATIONS/RISK FACTORS Facial nerve palsy including Bell's palsy, proptosis, reduced consciousness (e.g. intensive care admission or general anaesthesia), ectropion, exophthalmos, poor Bell's phenomenon.

EPIDEMIOLOGY Common in the conditions above.

HISTORY Dry eye/burning/irritation, epiphoria. Ask about history of thyroid disease (as a cause of exophthalmos).

EXAMINATION Lagophthalmos, conjunctival injection, superficial punctate epithelial erosions on the corneal surface. Cranial nerve examination with particular reference to CNVII function

PATHOLOGY/PATHOGENESIS
• Incomplete eye closure predisposes to the interpalprebal corneal surface being exposed to the environment and not being protected by protective blinking and the barrier function of the eyelid.
• The Bell's phenomenon causes the eyeball to turn upwards on eye closure. If defective, the cornea is at greater risk from lagophthalmos.

INVESTIGATIONS Imaging or other investigation may be indicated dependant on aetiology, for example in unexplained CNVII palsy or exophthalmos.

MANAGEMENT
• *Medical:* Regular tear substitutes or ointments. Patients who are in ITU, or are undergoing general anaesthetic, may have their eyelids closed temporally with tape as a preventative measure. Botulinium induced temporary ptosis can be considered in some patients.
• *Surgical:* Tarsorraphy (partial surgical closure of the eyelid, can be temporary). Upper eyelid gold weight insertion.

COMPLICATIONS Infectious keratitis.

PROGNOSIS May require lifelong lubricants if there is not a correctable underlying cause.

Eye trauma ▶

- Ocular injury can be severe and sight threatening but should not be taken out of context of other injuries that may be life-threatening in trauma cases. Chemical Injury is featured in an earlier chapter.
- Full history and examination should be performed including both eyes. Careful documentation is essential, especially for medicolegal purposes.
- Tetanus status should be ascertained.

Eyelid lacerations/cuts
Depth of the lesion is important to assess in case of injury to the globe. Any lesions that include the canaliculi or eyelid margins require repair by an experience ophthalmic surgeon.

Corneal foreign bodies
Patients will normally recall the instant a foreign body enters the eye (a high index of suspicion for intraocular foreign body if high velocity). The foreign body can be removed under slit lamp visualization after instillation of a topical anaesthetic. The upper eyelid should be everted to check for any foreign material. A five-day course of three times a day chloramphenicol ointment can help prevent secondary infection. Rust rings can form if the foreign body is metallic and will require removal by an ophthalmologist.

Corneal abrasion
Very painful, these superficial corneal injuries may be due to minor trauma or the entry of particulate matter onto the ocular surface. Examination with fluorescein stain reveals defects in the corneal epithelium. Once any foreign matter, including from underneath the eyelids, has been removed, the abrasion should heal well with a five-day course of prophylactic chloramphenicol ointment.

Hyphaema
Trauma can cause blood to collect in the anterior chamber. This leads to the risk of glaucoma and corneal staining. It will need ophthalmological review for consideration of admission for treatment.

Iris mydriasis
Blunt injury to iris spincter can cause permanent iris dilation.

Lens subluxation/dislocation
Rupture of greater than 25% zonular fibres will lead to the lens becoming subluxed and appearing decentred. Lens dislocation results from complete disruption of zonular attachments.

Eye trauma ▶ (continued)
Vitreous haemorrhage
Trauma can lead to bleeding into the vitreous cavity. Clinically this may manifest as profoundly poor vision and an inability to obtain a view of the fundus.

Retinal detachment
Trauma can cause retinal detachment. See 'Retinal detachment', **p. 110**.

Traumatic optic neuropathy
Poor vision, defective colour vision and an RAPD, not explained by a retinal lesion may be due to traumatic optic neuropathy. Pallor of the optic nerve may take weeks to develop.

Globe rupture/penetrating eye injury
There is usually a history of severe head injury or assault. Suspect if history indicates a potentially penetrating injury. Penetration of foreign bodies should be ruled out by an ophthalmologist where there is a history of high velocity particles involved (e.g. grinding metal/hammering). There may be herniation of intraocular contents. CT may reveal such an injury when performed as part of the work-up for a severe head injury. A plastic eye shield (not pad) should be placed over the eye whilst ophthalmology review is urgently sought.

Orbital fractures
Orbital floor fracture is the most common orbital fracture. It can result from blunt trauma to the orbit (blow out fracture). There may be limited upgaze causing vertical diplopia, enophthalmos and anaesthesia in the distribution of the infraorbital nerve. Patients should be advised not to blow their nose. Orbital and facial CTs should be obtained. Maxillofacial and ophthalmology referrals should be made.

Retrobulbar haemorrhage
Tense eyelids, inability to open the eye, extensive sunconjunctival haemorrhage, proptosis, reduced vision and a RAPD may indicate retrobulbar haemorrhage. Urgent canthotomy and cantholysis should be performed. This should be performed immediately on clinical diagnosis and should not be delayed for imaging confirmation or review by an ophthalmologist.

Eye tumours ▶

These are rare even in ophthalmology clinics and are typically managed by tertiary referral centres.

Primary choroidal melanoma

The incidence of choroidal melanoma is 6 per million per year and this is the most common primary intraocular malignancy. This tumour arises from melanocytes within the choroid. Patients may complain of visual field defects, visual distortion and floaters. There can be systemic involvement from metastasis.

Secondary (metastatic) choroidal

Visual impairment due to a secondary choroidal tumour may rarely be a first presentation of bronchial carcinoma. In women, this may represent metastasis from breast cancer. Prognosis is poor as the tumour often presents late with established disease.

Retinal haemangioma

This is a tumour associated with Von Hippel-Lindau disease. Patients present at a young age and examination of the fundus will reveal well-defined red oval regions on retina.

Ocular non-Hodgkin lymphoma

This is the most common type of ocular lymphoma and can be intraocular or orbital. A third of cases are associated with systemic lymphoma. Presentation can be with floaters, distorted vision or a red eye. Primary intraocular lymphoma is a form of primary central nervous system lymphoma that can present with focal neurological deficit, seizures or signs of raised intracranial pressure. This form has a very poor prognosis.

Giant cell arteritis (GCA)▶ (including Wegener's granulomatosis and Behçet's disease)

DEFINITION Vasculitis affecting medium and large-sized arteries.

AETIOLOGY Unknown. Some studies suggest an infectious origin based upon epidemiological observations.

ASSOCIATIONS/RISK FACTORS Increased age (rarely occurs under the age of 55); average age of onset is 70 years. Race – more common in Caucasians. Twice as common in women than men. Smoking. 50% of cases have associated polymyalgia rheumatica (PMR). There is association with human leukocyte antigens (HLA); DRB1, DRA4, DR3 and complement factor H polymorphisms.

EPIDEMIOLOGY
Incidence estimated at 2/100 000 in patients in their 60s.

HISTORY
• *Ocular:* permanent monocular visual loss, transient descending curtain like monocular visual loss (amaurosis fugax), diplopia, ocular pain.
• *Systemic:* scalp tenderness (for example, on combing the hair, laying their head on a pillow), headache, PMR (pain and stiffness in proximal muscles, usually the shoulders), fatigue, malaise, weight loss, fevers, jaw claudication, anorexia.

EXAMINATION
• Temporal artery tenderness/prominance/pulsatility (pulsatility initially present but can become nonpulsatile).
• Visual fields, pupil check for RAPD, intraocular pressures, eye movements (for cranial nerve palsies), fundus examination for signs of acute anterior ischaemic optic neuropathy (AAION); optic disc swelling/late disc pallor/disc haemorrhage/cotton wool spots. AAION may result in very poor visual acuity (may be NPL). Auscultation – carotid bruit, aortic regurgitation (may be present in aortic aneurysm).

PATHOLOGY/PATHOGENESIS
• Granulomatous inflammation of medium and large-sized arteries. There is segmental involvement of the vessels. Epitheloid and giant cells are present histologically. There is fibrosis of the intima and the internal elastic lamina becomes fragmented.
• These inflammatory changes cause obstruction of the vessel's lumen or precipitate thrombosis. This can lead to ischaemia of the structures supplied by the vessel. For example, obstruction of the blood supply to the short posterior ciliary arteries causes ischaemia of the optic nerve head leading to AAION. This is the most common cause of visual loss in GCA. As the risk of thromboembolization is increased also, central retinal artery occlusion (CRAO) can occur. Cotton wool spots can occur due to microemboli.

Giant cell arteritis (GCA)▶ (including Wegener's granulomatosis and Behçet's disease) (continued)

INVESTIGATIONS Raised ESR, CRP. Raised platelets. Temporal artery biopsy (may not be conclusive due to 'skip lesions'). Artery ultrasound (for halo sign).

MANAGEMENT
- Immediate high dose steroids (e.g. oral prednisolone 60 mg OD) without delay. The aim is to prevent contralateral loss of vision.
- Urgent rheumatology referral is warranted.
- Steroids may be required for up to two years with doses based on monitoring of symptoms and ESR.

COMPLICATIONS Permanent visual loss. Stroke, dissecting aneurysm, renal failure, angina pectoris, myocardial infarction, congestive cardiac failure.

PROGNOSIS The condition can have a protracted course, lasting for two years in cases. Restoration/preservation of visual function is dependent on the rapidity of steroid administration. Vision rarely improves if there is AAION or CRAO. If untreated, the fellow eye will be affected in almost all cases.

Wegener's granulomatosis

This is a vasculitis that affects small and medium sized vessels of any organ. It typically affects the nose, lungs and kidneys. Common clinical features include frequent nose bleeds, saddle nose deformity due to perforation of the nasal septum, pulmonary haemorrhage and haemoptysis, glomerulonephritis and chronic renal failure. Raised cytoplasmic ANCA levels can support diagnosis. Biopsy will reveal granulomatous inflammation. Initial treatment is with corticosteroids. There can be ocular inflammation causing features such as retinal artery occlusion, episcleritis, uveitis, proptosis and necrotizing scleritis with corneal infiltrates.

Behçet's disease

A triad of recurrent oral ulcers, genital ulcers and uveitis characterize this chronic, multisystem inflammatory disorder. Vasculitis of small and large vessels can occur which can cause fatal aneurysms of the pulmonary arterial tree. However, pathological inflammation of veins is a main cause of clinical symptoms. Other ocular features include retinal capillary leakage and retinal vein occlusions.

Glaucoma, acute primary angle-closure ▶

DEFINITION An optic neuropathy caused by an acute rise in intraocular pressure (IOP) secondary to closure of the irido-corneal angle. This is an ophthalmic emergency.

AETIOLOGY Aqueous fluid normally flows from the posterior chamber, though the pupil into the anterior chamber, and then out through the trabecular meshwork which is located between angle formed by the peripheral iris and the cornea. Forward movement of the iris can block this angle and thus prevent drainage of the fluid leading to an acute rise in IOP.

ASSOCIATIONS/RISK FACTORS Hypermetropia (which is often characterized by eyes with crowded structures owing to their relatively small size), increased age, females affected more commonly than males (4:1), family history, shallow anterior chamber. Rarely complicates pharmacological pupil dilation in at risk individuals.

EPIDEMIOLOGY Common in Eskimos and Asians. Uncommon in Blacks.

HISTORY Severe eye pain, nausea, vomiting, (may misleadingly present as an acute abdomen), headache, red eye, rainbow halos around lights, decreased vision. There may be a preceding history of intermittent blurred vision, and halos around lights, for example after an evening in a dark environment, due to transient closure of the irido-corneal angle caused by pupil dilation.

EXAMINATION Poor visual acuity, red eye (ciliary flush), cloudy cornea (secondary to corneal oedema), fixed and mid-dilated oval shaped pupil, eye that is stone hard on palpation, shallow anterior chamber, RAPD if optic nerve damage has occurred.

PATHOLOGY/PATHOGENESIS
- The posterior iris becomes appositional with the anterior lens. This causes a block of aqueous outflow through the pupil. There is a resultant increase in pressure of the posterior chamber relative to the anterior chamber which causes bulging forward of the peripheral iris; leading it to block the angle as described above.
- The acute and significant rise in IOP damages ocular structures. The corneal endothelial pump, which maintains hydration and subsequently clarity of the cornea, ceases to function causing corneal oedema. The pressure rise also causes damage to the optic nerve which can be permanent and blinding.
- Age is a risk factor because the lens, as it develops cataract, increases in size thus promoting pupil block.

Glaucoma, acute primary angle-closure ▶
(continued)

INVESTIGATIONS N/A – intraocular pressure assessment, slit lamp examination and gonioscopy (examination of the irido-corneal angle using a contact lens) will be performed by an ophthalmologist.

MANAGEMENT

* *Urgent referral to ophthalmology:* For assessment and immediate reduction of IOP with agents including parenteral/oral acetazolamide, topical pilocarpine, dexamethasone, timolol and iopidine. Peripheral laser iridotomy (PI) in the fellow eye is performed as an urgent prophylactic measure and is performed in the affected eye as soon as corneal clarity is restored.
* Cataract extraction and prophylactic PI can be performed in eyes that have narrow, and therefore potentially occludable angles.

COMPLICATIONS There is a risk of further pressure rise unless definitive PI is performed. Over 50% will develop acute angle closure glaucoma in the fellow eye if not prophylactically treated.

PROGNOSIS Severe attacks, especially if not promptly treated, can lead to irreversible damage to the optic nerve head and consequent blindness. There can be IOP rises over time due to damage sustained to the trabecular meshwork during the acute attack (a form of chronic open angle glaucoma). This necessitates long term follow-up.

Glaucoma, chronic open angle

DEFINITION A chronic and progressive condition that causes an optic neuropathy with characteristic visual field loss.

AETIOLOGY

- Glaucoma can exist in the presence of normal intraocular pressure (normal tension glaucoma). There can be raised intraocular pressure without signs of optic nerve damage (ocular hypertension).
- Raised intraocular pressure in primary open angle glaucoma is due to resistance, of unknown cause, of aqueous outflow through the drainage pathways.
- Secondary open angle glaucoma is due to a known aetiological factor causing restriction of aqueous outflow through the trabecular meshwork, for example inflammatory cells, blood cells (from a hyphaema), steroid use or pigment. Secondary causes may be related to trauma.

ASSOCIATIONS/RISK FACTORS Raised intraocular pressure, increased age, race - more severe and more common in Blacks, family history, diabetes mellitus, myopia, thin cornea, nocturnal hypotension, migraine, Raynaud's phenomenon.

EPIDEMIOLOGY The second most common cause of blindness in the world.

HISTORY Usually asymptomatic. Patient reported field loss (tunnel vision) only in severe late stage disease. Most are detected on routine examination at the optometrist or by screening those with a family history.

EXAMINATION Visual acuity, visual fields, RAPD (present in severe optic nerve damage), optic disc cupping/pallor/atrophy. Ophthalmologists will check intraocular pressure (IOP) by Goldmann applanation tonometry – pressure >21 mmHg is a risk factor for glaucoma.

PATHOLOGY/PATHOGENESIS The optic nerve axons in patients with glaucoma are susceptible to either direct pressure effects or ischaemia associated with impaired flow through the microvasculature supplying them. The retinal ganglion cells undergo apoptosis.

INVESTIGATIONS Automated visual field assessment, optic disc imaging, central corneal thickness. Blood glucose and BP (including 24 hour monitoring) if normal tension glaucoma suspected.

Glaucoma, chronic open angle (continued)

MANAGEMENT
- Needs referral to an ophthalmologist. Treatment of any underlying causes.
- Reduction of intraocular pressure, even in those with normal pressure, prevents glaucoma progression.
- *Medical:* IOP lowering agents – Topical B-Blockers **(contraindicated and potentially fatal in asthmatics!)**, prostaglandin analogues, carbonic anhydrase inhibitors, sympathomimetics.
- *Surgical:* In resistant and progressive cases; laser trabeculoplasty, surgical trabeculectomy.

COMPLICATIONS Severe visual field loss, blindness.

PROGNOSIS Regular monitoring and good control of IOP is often effective in preventing visual field loss.

Herpes zoster ophthalmicus (HZO) ▶

DEFINITION A reactivation of the varicella-zoster virus (VZV) involving the ophthalmic division of the trigeminal nerve.

AETIOLOGY VZV is a double-stranded DNA virus of the herpesviridae family. Primary infection manifests as chicken pox whereas secondary infection manifests as herpes zoster.

ASSOCIATIONS/RISK FACTORS Age (due to declining immunity to the virus), Immunosupressive therapy, HIV/Aids.

EPIDEMIOLOGY Incidence peaks in the 70s and above age group. Up to 20% of cases of herpes zoster involve the ophthalmic division of the trigeminal nerve.

HISTORY Prodrome/flu-like symptoms/fever; may precede cutaneous manifestations by a week. Patients may complain of neuralgia or later a rash affecting the forehead/upper eyelid/nose. Symptoms of eye pain or decreased vision should be elicited. The possibility of immunosuppression should be explored. Patients may be photophobic if there is uveitis.

EXAMINATION
- *Dermatomal rash distribution:* initially papules which turn into vesicles which develop into pustules. These lyse and crust over. There may be eyelid swelling and a red eye.
- *Hutchinson's sign:* rash affecting the tip of the nose. This is supplied by the nasal branch of the nasocillliary nerve which supplies the cornea so should raise suspicion of ocular involvement.
- *Visual acuity:* may be decreased in ocular involvement. RAPD – if there is optic neuritis (rare) or retinal necrosis.
- Corneal sensation may be impaired. Staining of the cornea may reveal epithelial defects. A keratitis may be present (best examined by an ophthalmologist). Also, an ophthalmologist will examine for uveitis and perform dilated fundus examination to check for retinal involvement.

PATHOLOGY/PATHOGENESIS Primary infection with VZV results in the virus entering the dorsal root ganglia where it lies dormant. Upon reactivation, which can occur decades after primary infection, virus particles traverse the ophthalmic division of the trigeminal nerve. Branches of this division (the nasociliary nerve) innervate the surface of the globe and the skin of the tip of the nose. Resulting inflammation can be destructive to surrounding tissues.

INVESTIGATIONS This is almost invariably a clinical diagnosis.

Herpes zoster ophthalmicus (HZO) ▶ (continued)

MANAGEMENT Systemic antiviral therapy, for example with oral acyclovir, can reduce disease duration and risk of complications if commenced early (within 72 hours of the onset of rash). Lubricants, topical acyclovir and prophylactic antibiotic ointment (e.g. chloramphenicol) may be needed for ocular surface disease. There is evidence emerging that a three-month course of low-dose amytriptiline can help prevent painful post-herpetic neuralgia.

COMPLICATIONS Microbial keratitis (secondary), raised intraocular pressure, retinal necrosis, uveitis, cranial nerve palsies, neurotrophic keratitis, post-herpetic neuralgia, cerebral vasculitis (see 'Keratitis, herpetic', p. 91).

PROGNOSIS Recurrence is common and half of patients may develop complications.

Horner's syndrome ▶

DEFINITION Interruption of the sympathetic innervation to the eye

AETIOLOGY
- Acquired – apical lung tumours (Pancoast's tumour), neck trauma/surgery, carotid artery aneurysm, carotid artery dissection, otitis media, brainstem lesions, diabetes mellitus.
- Congenital.

ASSOCIATIONS/RISK FACTORS Can be associated with migraine.

EPIDEMIOLOGY Dependent on the underlying cause.

HISTORY Droopy eyelid, Cosmetic concern (apparent enophthalmos).

EXAMINATION Ipsilateral – miosis, anisocoria (exacerbated in the dark by dilatation of the normal pupil). Anhydrosis of the ipsilateal half of the face (depending on level of lesion). Examine for signs of respiratory/central tumours. Congenital/long standing cases – lighter coloured iris. Intracranial pathology may be associated with cranial nerve signs.

PATHOLOGY/PATHOGENESIS Diverse pathology can affect sympathetic nerve supply to the eye because of the course of the nerve. It arises from the posterior hypothalamus and follows a course through ciliospinal centre and then the superior cervical ganglion, approaching the apex of the lung en route. It then ascends alongside the internal carotid artery and follows the path of the ophthalmic division of the trigeminal nerve within the cavernous sinus. The supply to the following is therefore interrupted hence the signs:

- Muller muscle – ptosis
- Dilator pupillae – miosis
- Skin supplied by ophthalmic division of the trigeminal nerve – anhydrosis
- Ciliary body – iris hypochromia

INVESTIGATIONS
- Depending on suspected underlying cause; FBC, blood glucose, chest X-ray, neuro/neck/spinal imaging.
- Pharmacological testing can be used to confirm that pupil signs are due to Horner's syndrome, for example:
  ○ Instillation of 4% cocaine into both eyes – dilation of a normal pupil. No dilation of a Horner's pupil. Cocaine is a noradrenaline (NA) re-uptake inhibitor that will lead to NA accumulation and dilation of the normal pupil. There is no sympathetic nerve supply hence no NA secreted in the Horner's eye so the pupil will remain constricted.

Horner's syndrome ▶ (continued)

MANAGEMENT Depends on underlying cause. Urgent referral to the appropriate specialty if concerns of malignancy. Congenital cases with cosmetic concern may benefit from ptosis repair.

COMPLICATIONS An underlying malignant cause can be fatal. Horner's syndrome can be a sign of rapidly fatal conditions such as carotid artery dissection.

PROGNOSIS Unlikely to resolve.

Hypertensive retinopathy

DEFINITION Retinopathy caused by microvascular damage induced by hypertension.

AETIOLOGY Most hypertension is idiopathic (essential hypertension). Malignant hypertension is a rare, severe and acute elevation of blood pressure.

ASSOCIATIONS/RISK FACTORS Smoking, obesity, high salt diets. Race – increased risk in Blacks. Increased age.

EPIDEMIOLOGY 25% of all adults have hypertension. Ophthalmic hypertensive changes present in 15% of patients with hypertension.

HISTORY
- A systemic history and examination should be performed as hypertension can cause life-threatening end-organ damage.
- Essential hypertension ; Often asymptomatic.
- Malignant hypertension – headache, scotoma, dimming of vision, diplopia.

EXAMINATION
- Arteriovenous nipping – hardened retinal arterioles impair flow through veins crossing them. This causes the apparent disappearance of the vein immediately adjacent to where the crossing takes place.
- Arteriolar narrowing. Flame haemorrhages. Cotton wool spots. Copper wiring; red-brown appearance of retinal arterioles. Silver wiring; opaque appearance of arterioles. Macular star; radially shaped collection of lipid deposits.
- Blood pressure in malignant hypertension; systolic > 200 mmHg and Diastolic >110
- Malignant hypertensive retinopathy may cause an optic neuropathy with papilloedema. There may be extensive flame shaped retinal haemorrhages.
- There are various classifications of hypertensive retinopathy, below is the modified Scheie Classification:
  - Grade 0: No changes
  - Grade 1: Barely detectable arterial narrowing
  - Grade 2: Obvious arterial narrowing with focal irregularities
  - Grade 3: Features of Grade 2 and retinal haemorrhages, cotton wool spots, exudates or retinal oedema
  - Grade 4: Features of Grade 3 and papilloedema

Hypertensive retinopathy (continued)

PATHOLOGY/PATHOGENESIS Hypertension induces atherosclerotic changes in the vasculature. Arteriolar vasoconstriction results from elevation of blood pressure. Venous occlusion leads to aneurysmal changes and subsequent haemorrhage due to rupture. In malignant hypertension, ischaemia of the optic nerve head, and resultant papilloedema, is due to constriction of the posterior ciliary arteries.

INVESTIGATIONS Blood pressure. Consideration of secondary causes.

MANAGEMENT
- Essential hypertension; manage with general practitioners: lifestyle changes – weight loss, smoking cessation, exercise. Antihypertensive therapy.
- Malignant hypertension – urgent medical admission for controlled blood pressure lowering.

COMPLICATIONS Retinal detachment. Anterior ischaemic optic neruopathy. Manifestations of end-organ damage – e.g. stroke, myocardial infarction, renal failure.

PROGNOSIS Hypertensive retinopathy with papilloedema is associated with a high risk of stroke and potentially irreversible visual loss.

Keratitis, bacterial ▶

DEFINITION Inflammation of the cornea caused by bacterial infection.

AETIOLOGY Common causative organisms include *Pseudomonas aeruginosa*, *Staphyloccus aureus*, *Staphylococcus epidermidis*, *Streptococcus pyogenes*, *Streptococcus pneumoniae*, Enterobacter. Viruses, protozoa (e.g. acanthamoeba from tap water contaminated contact lenses), and fungi (from organic contamination) can cause infectious keratitis. Microsporidia is a fungal cause to be considered in HIV patients.

ASSOCIATIONS/RISK FACTORS
• Contact lens wear (pseudomonal infection most likely in such cases).
• Concurrent ocular surface disease such as dry eye, corneal anaesthesia, severe allergic eye disease, eyelid abnormalities. Immunosuppression, Vitamin A deficiency, trauma.

EPIDEMIOLOGY Bacterial keratitis is the most common cause of infectious keratitis. It is rare in the absence of a predisposing factor such as contact lens wear or trauma. In contact lens wearers a sterile keratitis may occur.

HISTORY Pain, sensation of foreign body, photophobia, discharge, blurred vision.

EXAMINATION Red (injected) conjunctiva, epithelial defect/ulcer (staining with fluorescein dye reveals a bright green defect when observed under the illumination of a blue light), stromal opacity (infiltrate), hypopyon (collection of pus in the anterior chamber if severe).

PATHOLOGY A normal corneal epithelium can be penetrated by some bacteria such as *Neisseria gonorrhoaea* and *Haemophilus Influenzae*. Most commonly, bacterial pathogens enter the corneal stroma through defects in the corneal epithelium. Matrix metalloproteinases, secreted by inflammatory cells, and proteases secreted by the pathogen, cause breakdown of the extracellular matrix. This further disrupts the barrier function of the cornea which can lead to corneal perforation.

INVESTIGATIONS *Microbiology:* Corneal scrapes need to be taken for gram staining, culture and antibiotic sensitivity by an ophthalmologist. The culture media used should include blood agar, chocolate agar, non- and cooked meat broth. Non-nutrient agar seeded with E Coli is used for the culture of acanthamoeba. Endophthalmitis should be excluded by ultrasound if corneal opacity impairs a full examination.

Keratitis, bacterial ▶ (continued)

MANAGEMENT Topical, broad spectrum antibiotics, e.g. fluorquinolone initally hourly, including overnight if indicated. Use of cyclopegic drops aid comfort. Review is important in order to check for progression and to adjust for antibiotic sensitivities if appropriate. Oral antibiotics are indicated in cases of threatened or actual corneal perforation. Caution and adherence to guidelines govern the use of topical steroids in the healing phase.

COMPLICATIONS Corneal ulceration may progress to perforation which can precipitate endophthalmitis. Scarring can lead to irregular astigmatism and reduced vision. Severe inflammation can lead to secondary cataract.

PROGNOSIS Corneal scarring or perforation may require surgical treatment, e.g. keratoplasty. Lens opacification may warrant cataract extraction. Endophthalmitis can cause permanent sight loss.

Keratitis, herpetic ▶

DEFINITION Inflammation of the cornea caused by viral infection.

AETIOLOGY Causative organisms include herpes simplex virus (HSV) and varicella-zoster virus (VZV), HSV is a double-stranded DNA virus. There are two serotypes; 1 typically affects the oropharynx region and 2 affects the genital area. However, each virus can affect either area. VZV causes both chicken pox and shingles.

ASSOCIATIONS/RISK FACTORS Previous viral infection (primary infection), herpes zoster ophthalmicus, immunosupression, diabetes mellitus, trauma. Stress, hormonal change or UV light may trigger reactivations.

EPIDEMIOLOGY Most cases occur in adulthood. Herpetic eye disease is a major cause of blindness due to corneal pathology.

HISTORY Painful eye, foreign body sensation, photophobia, epiphora, redness, reduced vision. There may have been a viral prodrome or vesicular rash around the eyelids. Previous episodes (patients can experience hundreds of HSV reactivations over their lifetime).

EXAMINATION
• There may be eyelid skin involvement or conjunctivitis. In VZV reactivation there is usually a preceding dermatomal rash. Patients may be systemically unwell in VZV reactivation and must be assessed and treated appropriately.
• Cornea – there may be reduced corneal sensation. HSV and VZV can cause an epithelial keratitis in the early stages of reactivation. Stromal infection is rare and in HSV can be necrotizing.
• HSV – initially stellate patterns of staining revealed by fluorescein. These develop into branch like linear patterns (dendritic lesions) with terminal buds.
• VZV epithelial keratitis may appear similar but on close slip lamp examination there are no terminal buds and the dendritic patterns are often smaller. Later stages of corneal involvement may manifest as a nummular keratitis (fine subepithelial deposits surrounded by hazy stromal areas).
• Ophthalmologists will examine for any increase in intraocular pressure, uveitis or retinitis that may be present.

PATHOLOGY Primary infection with HSV is very common and most often subclinical. Primary infection results in latent infection as the virus ascends sensory trigeminal nerve axons. Clinical reactivation results from transport of the virus to peripheral nerve endings and viral replication. VZV reactivation in the ophthalmic branch of the trigeminal nerve causes herpes zoster ophthalmicus (HZO) and nasociliary branch involvement will affect the cornea (see HZO, **p. 83**).

Keratitis, herpetic ▶ (continued)

INVESTIGATIONS Diagnosis is clinical. Confirmatory tests are rarely required but include; Enzyme-linked immunosorbent assay, viral culture or microscopy and staining of corneal scrapings.

MANAGEMENT
- There is evidence that early initiation of oral Aciclovir in HSV reactivation can reduce future recurrence and reduce rates of stromal keratitis. Patients with frequent recurrences may require long-term prophylaxis with oral aciclovir.
- Initiation of oral acyclovir in VZV infection (ideally within 72 hours of rash onset) can reduce duration and sequelae of the disease. Topical aciclovir ointment is commonly used in acute epithelial disease. Bacterial prophylaxis with chloramphenicol ointment is employed by some.

COMPLICATIONS Necrotizing stromal keratitis; a rare complication of HSV keratitis. Secondary bacterial infection. Steroid-use associated cataract or glaucoma. Neurotrophic ulceration. Post-herpetic neuralgia can affect a significant proportion of patients.

PROGNOSIS Corneal scarring can affect visual prognosis.

Keratoconjunctivitis sicca

DEFINITION Dry eye.

AETIOLOGY Reduced aqueous tear production and/or increased tear evaporation.

ASSOCIATIONS/RISK FACTORS Systemic autoimmune disease, Sjögren's syndrome, contact lens wear, Bell's palsy, Parkinson's disease, cicatrising conjunctival disorders (e.g. Trachoma), defective tearing reflex (e.g. after laser refractive surgery), Vitamin A deficiency.

EPIDEMIOLOGY Very common.

HISTORY
- Irritation/dryness/burning of the eyes. Red eye, mild photophobia, foreign body sensation. Episodes of reflex epiphora.
- Cold weather, air conditioning and central heating can exacerbate symptoms as can prolonged reading or computer use.
- Sjögren's syndrome - dry mouth

EXAMINATION Conjunctival hyperaemia, corneal erosions (superficial punctate epithelial erosions), low tear film height and break-up time. Schirmer test – measure the progression of wetting of a strip of filter paper that has had its tip placed under the lower eyelid. A length of <5 mm of progression in 5 minutes is abnormal.

PATHOLOGY/PATHOGENESIS
- Sjogren's syndrome – autoimmune lymphocytic infiltration of exocrine glands that leads to reduced secretion of the aqueous component of tears.
- Reflex tearing relies on corneal sensation which is reduced in contact lens wear or trigeminal nerve defects.
- The eyelids are responsible for forming the intricately layered tear film and defects, such as ectropion, impair this and lead to abnormal tear film evaporation.
- Rosacea causes abnormality of the meibomian glands and increased evaporation of tears due to a defective oily tear layer.
- Reduced blinking, as in cases of Parkinson's disease, or when using computer screens, leads to evaporative drying.

INVESTIGATIONS
- Sjogren's syndrome – may be proven by labial biopsy. Suspicion of underlying systemic autoimmune disease may require rheumatology referral and blood testing for anti-nuclear antibody (ANA) and rheumatoid factor (RF).
- Ophthalmologists can employ a plethora of special examination techniques and staining methods to test for signs of keratoconjunctivitis sicca.

Keratoconjunctivitis sicca (continued)

MANAGEMENT
- *Patient education:* management is based on symptom control and prevention of progression.
- *Tear substitutes:* a multitude are available, for example carboxymethylcellulose, carbomer.
- *Punctal occlusion:* ophthalmologists may occlude the lacrimal punctae (and therefore reduce tear drainage) temporarily or permanently, using plugs or cautery respectively.
- *Anti-inflammatory agents:* may be employed in severe cases.

COMPLICATIONS Corneal ulceration, bacterial keratitis, corneal perforation.

PROGNOSIS Chronic and incurable in most cases.

Keratoconus

DEFINITION Corneal ectasia; progressive thinning and distortion of the cornea. The name arises from the conical distortion of the cornea in advanced cases.

AETIOLOGY Unknown

ASSOCIATIONS/RISK FACTORS Down's syndrome, eye rubbing and atopy, Turner's syndrome, Ehlers-Danlos, Marfan's syndrome, Leber's congenital amaurosis, osteogenesis imperfecta, retinitis pigmentosa, vernal keratoconjunctivitis.

EPIDEMIOLOGY Prevalence 1/2000. There is a positive family history in a small percentage of cases.

HISTORY Onset usually in puberty, asymmetric and progressive worsening of vision/increasing requirement to change glasses prescription (due to worsening myopia and astigmatism), glare, monocular diplopia. Intolerance of contact lenses.

EXAMINATION Munson's sign – on down gaze the protruding cornea causes bulging forward of the lower eyelid. 'Oil-droplet' red reflex seen with direct ophthalmoscopy at a distance of about 30 cm. Rizutti's sign – on shining a penlight from the temporal aspect a conical reflection can be seen on the nasal cornea. Corneal scarring. Slit lamp – deep stromal lines (Vogt lines), Fleischer's ring (epithelial iron deposits).

PATHOLOGY/PATHOGENESIS The precise curvature of the cornea plays a significant role in focusing light on the retina. There is thinning of the stroma and central protrusion of the cornea in Keratoconus leading to distorted focus. It is postulated that abnormally increased protease activity breaks down the collagen crosslinks that maintain the corneal stroma.

INVESTIGATIONS Corneal thickness, corneal topography. Tests for co-existing genetic conditions may be indicated.

MANAGEMENT
- Corrective glasses in early cases. Rigid contact lenses can correct greater degrees of refractive error.
- *Surgical:* Keratoplasty (corneal grafting). Riboflavin application and activation by UV light causes new crosslinks to form within the stroma thus maintain its integrity. This is a novel treatment and has been shown to prevent progression of keratoconus in some studies. Intrastromal ring segments are being implanted with success in some patients.

Keratoconus (continued)

COMPLICATIONS Acute corneal hydrops – there is rupture of descemet's membrane allowing aqueous fluid into the cornea. It is associated with a sudden onset of reduced visual acuity, tearing and discomfort.

PROGNOSIS Bilateral keratoconus will develop in half of those with only one affected eye on presentation. There is variation in the timeline of progression. Most can be effectively treated.

Lid lumps, basal cell carcinoma

DEFINITION A malignant and slow growing tumour of basal cells in the epidermis of the skin.

AETIOLOGY Chronic exposure to sunlight.

ASSOCIATIONS/RISK FACTORS Fair skin, xeroderma pigmentosum, immunosupression, Gorlin's syndrome (autosomal dominant condition associated with multiple BCCs, hypertelorism, scoliosis, pectus excavatum and palmar pits).

EPIDEMIOLOGY >90% of malignant eyelid tumours are basal cell carcinomas.

HISTORY Painless nodule or a nonhealing ulcer that bleeds easily. Normally slowly growing for months or years.

EXAMINATION Most occur on the lower eyelid. Numerous clinical forms of BCC exist, however, three particular forms predominate on the eyelid:

- *Nodular:* firm nodule with pearly appearance. Fine telangiectasia may be visible.
- *Noduloulcerative (rodent ulcer):* as for nodular BCC but with central ulceration and crusting. Characteristically raised, rolled pearly edges. Prominent telangiectasia also feature.
- *Sclerosing (morphoeic):* indurated, waxy scar-like plaque. The edges are poorly defined. Palpation may reveal a more extensive lesion than initial inspection.

PATHOLOGY Histology – groups of small, basophilic epithelial cells derived from pluripotent basal cells. BCCs are locally invasive but rarely metastasize.

INVESTIGATIONS Histology confirms diagnosis following biopsy.

MANAGEMENT
- *Surgical excision:* treatment of choice. Various techniques can be employed including Moh's micrographic surgery (associated with lower recurrence rates, especially for recurrent tumours).
- *Cryotherapy:* uses the destructive effects of the extremely cold temperatures ($-20\,°C$) that can be attained by the use of liquid nitrogen.
- *Radiotherapy:* can be used as an alternative for lower risk lesions but is associated with higher recurrence rates and complications such as keratitis and dry eyes.

Lid lumps, basal cell carcinoma (continued)

COMPLICATIONS If untreated, lesions enlarge and are locally destructive. They can reoccur if inadequately treated.

PROGNOSIS There is an excellent cure rate following complete excision (>95% at 5 years).

Lid lumps, chalazion

DEFINITION Chronic inflammatory granuloma caused by retention of tarsal meibomian gland secretions.

AETIOLOGY The openings of the oil-producing meibomian glands within the tarsal plates of the upper and lower eyelids become plugged. This leads to the retention of sebum within the tarsus and eyelid soft tissue, causing an inflammatory reaction.

ASSOCIATIONS/RISK FACTORS Acne rosacea, chronic blepharitis.

EPIDEMIOLOGY Commonly seen in clinical practice. More frequently in adults. Occurs more commonly on the upper eyelid.

HISTORY Acute tender eyelid swelling often resolving to reveal a painless nodule on the eyelid. Patients may report a sensation of heaviness. Cosmetic concerns often prompt presentation to a doctor. Rarely, pressure from the chalazion can cause astigmatism and blurred vision.

EXAMINATION Nodule within the tarsal place. Non-tender. The underlying conjunctiva may appear erythematous.

PATHOLOGY/PATHOGENESIS The release of sebum induces a chronic inflammatory reaction comprising of granulation tissue rich in multinucleated giant cells.

INVESTIGATIONS If there is any suspicion of malignancy, or if the chalazion is recurrent after previous incision, the lesion should be biopsied for histological study to exclude sebaceous gland carcinoma.

MANAGEMENT May resolve with no treatment. Hot compresses and eyelid hygiene can lead to resolution of the lesion. Patients should be instructed to dip the end of a cotton bud into hot water and massage the tip of the bud into the lump to help melt and release the oils. Incision and curettage, often as an outpatient procedure, is the main surgical intervention employed. Intralesional steroid injection is sometimes indicated.

COMPLICATIONS Rupture of a chalazion can occur on either of the eyelid surfaces. This may be seen on the conjunctival surface as a granuloma. Secondary infection of a chalazion, with organisms such as *Staphylococcus aureus,* causes an internal hordeolum.

PROGNOSIS One-third to half resolve spontaneously without treatment. Incision and curettage is 95% successful. Effective treatment of blepharitis is preventative.

Lid lumps, other (benign)
Cyst of Zeiss
Cyst on the margin of the eyelid filled with the yellowish secretion of
sebaceous glands. Removal would be for cosmesis.

Cyst of Moll
Cyst on the margin of the eyelid filled with the translucent secretion of
sweat glands. Removal would be for cosmesis.

Molluscum contagiosum
Dome-shaped umbilicated papule, pearly or flesh coloured. They are
caused by a DNA pox virus. They may occur in clusters and can be
treated by excision. Viral shedding can cause a chronic follicular
conjunctivitis.

Stye (external hordeolum)
Abscess of an eyelash follicle. This will be tender and have a pointed
head of pus. They can be treated with chloramphenicol ointment and
hot compresses.

Squamous cell papilloma
These are multilobar in appearance and pedunculated. Most often
these are benign but should be excised for histological analysis if they
are large or have features suspicious of malignancy.

Xanthelasma
Yellow lipid containing plaque, often located on the nasal sides of the
eyelids. They can indicate hypercholesterolaemia which should be
investigated and managed. Removal would be cosmetic.

Lid lumps, other (malignant)
Note on malignancy
The eyelid skin, like skin anywhere else on the body, is susceptible to malignancy so any lesions must be evaluated with this in mind. Features that should raise suspicion include:

- Rapid growth
- Change in pigmentation
- Irregular borders
- Bleeding
- Associated eyelash loss
- Systemic features
- Previous history of skin cancers

Squamous cell carcinoma (SCC)
An aggressive tumour in which metastasis is common. They may be indistinguishable from other tumours and may arise *de novo* from pre-existing tumours. They may be en plaque, papular or nodular form, with crusting and erosion. They may have an ulcerated or necrotic base with everted borders but are less likely to feature pearly edges and surface telangiectasia than BCC. In situ SCC can present as 'Cutenous Horns' which are hornlike projections of keratin. Urgent referral is needed.

Melanoma
A nodule or plaque of new or changing pigmentation should raise suspicion of this. The borders of such a lesion may be irregular. There is often diagnostic difficulty because half of eyelid melanomas are not pigmented. Urgent referral is needed.

Merkel cell carcinoma
This is a highly malignant tumour that arises from a specialized epithelial cell; the merkel cell. It is rare and presents as a rapidly growing dome shaped papule or nodule. It may appear violet, red or pink. Urgent referral is needed and recurrence is high despite excision. Prognosis is poor and 50% of patients have metastatic spread at presentation.

Keratocanthoma
This is rare and presents as a rapidly growing lesion (can grow 2 cm in weeks). It is dome-shaped with erythema and a central keratotic plug. Clinical examination cannot rule out SCC therefore urgent referral is required for excision.

Migraine

DEFINITION Recurrent headache disorder.

AETIOLOGY Family history. Rarely genetic disorders such as familial hemiplegic migraine or mitochondrial disorders such as CADASIL (cerebral autosomal dominant arteriopathy with subcortical infarcts and leukoencephalopathy). Hormonal contraceptives.

ASSOCIATIONS/RISK FACTORS There is an increased risk of stroke or cardiovascular disease in patients.

EPIDEMIOLOGY Prevalence around 10%. 75% of sufferers are women.

HISTORY
- *Classic migraine (migraine with aura):* visual aura; flashes/patterns/scotoma/zig-zag lines in vision. Arcs of missing vision. Usually bilateral (this will require very careful history taking to elicit) and lasting around 15 minutes then followed by severe throbbing headache. Other types of aura can occur and include transient weakness or aphasia.
- *Migraine without aura:* vague prodromal visual symptoms may occur but the predominant symptoms are headache and nausea.
- *Basillar migraine:* Hemianopia, vertigo, diplopia, ataxia; can occur with or without subsequent headache.
- Rare forms of migraine include hemiparetic migraine or ophthalmoplegic migraine.
- Elicit any triggering features – environment/foods

EXAMINATION Neurological signs corresponding to the above may be present. Causes such as stroke, transient ischaemic attacks, meningitis and subarachnoid haemorrhages can present with similar signs and symptoms so must be included within the differential, especially upon a first presentation. As migraine sufferers are at increased risk of thromboembolic events one must exclude this in atypical migraine presentations. Rarely, intracranial space occupying lesions can present with migraine like symptoms.

PATHOLOGY/PATHOGENESIS This is not known with certainty. Current theory relates neuron hypersensitivity to altered cerebral perfusion and function.

INVESTIGATIONS Typical symptoms can be diagnostic however neuroimaging may be required to rule out sinister causes.

MANAGEMENT Avoidance of triggers. Analgesics – such as aspirin or paracetamol. 5HT1B/1D agonists such as sumatriptan can be effective during an attack. As prophylaxis in frequently recurring migraines beta blockers, antidepressants and anticonvulsants can be effective.

Migraine (continued)

COMPLICATIONS Increased risk of stroke, especially in women who have migraine with aura and are on the combined oral contraceptive pill.

PROGNOSIS Trigger avoidance rarely prevents all attacks. Migraine is a recurrent problem that is a drain to the UK economy due to loss of production of >£200 million pounds a year.

Multiple sclerosis (MS)

DEFINITION CNS disorder with neurological impairment. Clinical features are disseminated in time and space.

AETIOLOGY Unknown. The incidence is lowest in equatorial regions. There is a 20% concordance rate between monozygotic twins. Such observations have led to the speculation that genetic factors combined with environmental factors are important in the aetiology.

ASSOCIATIONS/RISK FACTORS Some association with HLA-DRB1.

EPIDEMIOLOGY Prevalence 50/100 000. The prevalence reduces significantly at latitudes approaching the equator.

HISTORY
- CNS lesions cause neurological symptoms that are characteristically disseminated in time and space. For example, a presentation may be with visual disturbance. This may resolve and a subsequent presentation may be with a weakness of a limb.
- Optic neuritis – may be an initial presentation (sometimes preceding onset and diagnosis of MS by years); causing pain on eye movement (typically unilateral), blurring of vision, central vision loss.
- Symptoms are wide-ranging due to wide ranging possible loci of lesions which can occur concurrently. For example there may be weakness, paresthesia, gait disturbance, brain-stem or cerebellar symptoms. There may also be autonomic dysfunction. Mood-related symptoms such as depression or euphoria can occur.
- Uthoff's phenomenon describes the worsening of symptoms with increases in body temperature (for example with fever or whilst taking a hot bath). Relapses can be induced by stress.

EXAMINATION
- Optic neuritis – papillitis if the lesion involves the optic nerve head. Retrobulbar optic neuritis will not manifest with this sign. Reduced visual acuity. Red desaturation (a bright red coloured target will appear dull in appearance compared to its appearance in the unaffected eye). There will be a RAPD. Occasionally colour vision defects and scotomata can persist. The optic disc will become pale over time due to optic atrophy.
- A full neurological examination needs to be performed to determine the extent of neurological deficit.

Multiple sclerosis (MS) (continued)

PATHOLOGY/PATHOGENESIS

- Active inflammatory lesions known as plaques are associated with demyelination in the CNS. CD4 T-cells mediate an immune response against myelin of the brain. Perivenular infiltration of lymphocytes and monocytes occurs and these cells accumulate leading to plaques of demyelination forming.
- A plaque can resolve with re-myelination and therefore CNS dysfunction can be reversible. However, permanent axonal destruction can occur in severe disease.

INVESTIGATIONS MRI reveals plaques. Electrophysiological tests, such as visual evoked responses, will be abnormal if there has been an episode of optic neuropathy. Lumbar puncture.

MANAGEMENT With neurologist support. IV Steroids can reduce the duration of relapses. Beta-interferon can reduce relapse rates. Rehabilitation and palliation are often required as disease progresses.

COMPLICATIONS Permanent disability. Dementia. Death.

PROGNOSIS There are various patterns of the condition that reflect the different forms:

- Relapsing and remitting: 80% – episodes of CNS features with complete or partial remission, followed by further relapses.
- Primary progressive: 10% – gradual clinical decline from onset with plateaus (during which there is no progression) but no periods of remission.
- Secondary progressive: 10% – pattern corresponding to an initial relapsing and remitting course that subsequently follows a primary progressive like pattern.
- Fulminant – rapid progression and deterioration over months with no remission.

Pinguecula

DEFINITION Benign conjunctival degeneration.

AETIOLOGY Cumulative UV damage

ASSOCIATIONS/RISK FACTORS Sun exposure/tropical climates.

EPIDEMIOLOGY Very common. Typically found in those over 40 years of age.

HISTORY Cosmetic concern, dry eye symptoms, irritation.

EXAMINATION Yellow/white growth on the conjunctiva adjacent to the limbus. There is no extension over the cornea. Most often occur around the nasal limbus.

PATHOLOGY/PATHOGENESIS UV mediated elastoid degeneration of conjunctival collagen fibres. This degeneration can progress to calcification.

INVESTIGATIONS None.

MANAGEMENT Tear substitutes to relieve irritation. Rarely, surgical excision may be indicated for cosmesis.

COMPLICATIONS This is a benign condition. Pingueculitis, an acute inflammation of the Pinguecula, can occur and may require a short course of topical steroids.

PROGNOSIS Slow enlargement can occur, the lesions may be bilateral.

Posterior vitreous detachment (PVD)

DEFINITION Detachment of the posterior vitreous from the retina.

AETIOLOGY Vitreous degeneration, a process that begins in adolescence, results in liquefaction of the vitreous. The vitreous is only weakly bound to the most of the posterior retina and such degeneration of the vitreous causes traction and subsequent separation of the vitreous from the retina. The liquefied vitreous can enter the potential space between retina and vitreous precipitating vitreous detachment which is exacerbated by eye movements.

ASSOCIATIONS/RISK FACTORS 10% or more of symptomatic PVDs are associated with a retinal tear or vitreous haemorrhage. Increased age, high myopia/myopia, ocular trauma, cataract extraction, uveitis, connective tissue disorders.

EPIDEMIOLOGY Some studies report a prevalence of greater than 50% amongst the elderly. It is rare in those under 40 with emmetropic eyes.

HISTORY Persistent flashes; commonly temporal, floaters, symptoms worse with eye movements. May be assymptomatic.

EXAMINATION Visual fields. Examination will need to be performed by an ophthalmologist. Slit lamp examination – may reveal a Weiss ring or haemorrhage. The peripheral retina must be examined to rule out retinal tears/detachments. A PVD may be present in the contralateral eye also.

PATHOLOGY/PATHOGENESIS It is thought that liquefaction of vitreous is caused by light mediated generation of free radicals that can disrupt cross links between collagen and hyaluronic acid. This is characterized by the appearance of liquid filled cavities within the vitreous. Over time the delicate gel like structure of the vitreous is prone to collapse.

INVESTIGATIONS B-Scan ultrasonography is indicated if the peripheral fundal view is impaired.

MANAGEMENT If there is no detachment reassurance can be given with a retinal detachment warning – i.e. urgent attention should be sought if there are worsening/new floaters/flashes or a curtain-like loss of visual field.

COMPLICATIONS Vitreous haemorrhage, retinal tears/detachment.

PROGNOSIS Many have no serious consequence and floaters become unnoticeable to patients but retinal tears can develop within weeks of a PVD.

Pterygium

DEFINITION Abnormal wing shaped growth of degenerative conjunctival tissue arising from the limbal conjunctiva and extending onto the cornea.

AETIOLOGY Chronic exposure to UV light.

ASSOCIATIONS/RISK FACTORS Chronic sun exposure/dry climates.

EPIDEMIOLOGY More common in those with outdoor lifestyles or those living in equatorial regions.

HISTORY Concerning cosmetic appearance, reduced vision, ocular irritation (will be greater in contact lens wearers).

EXAMINATION More frequently seen around the nasal limbus, hyperaemia (if inflamed). Slit Lamp-Stocker's line; Iron deposits (within the corneal epithelium) anterior to the advancing edge of the lesion.

PATHOLOGY/PATHOGENESIS Proliferation of the subepithelial fibrovascular component of the conjunctiva. This in-growth can cause destruction of Bowman's layer.

INVESTIGATIONS N/A.

MANAGEMENT Regular lubricant eye drops and occasional courses of topical anti-inflammatories. UV light avoidance (sunglasses) to prevent progression. Surgical excision may be indicated for cosmesis/impaired vision/recurrent inflammation.

COMPLICATIONS Astigmatism/obscuration of the visual axis, corneal scarring corneal perforation. Complications are rare.

PROGNOSIS Frequently follow an indolent course and do not require surgery. High recurrence rates after surgical excision have been reduced by conjunctival autografting.

Retinal artery occlusion ▶

DEFINITION There can be occlusion of the central retinal artery or one of its branches.

AETIOLOGY Atherosclerotic carotid artery disease is the most common cause. Rarely; giant cell arteritis, sickle cell disease, cardiac emboli. Infective; syphilis.

ASSOCIATIONS/RISK FACTORS Increased age, diabetes mellitus, hypertension, smoking, hypercholesterolaemia, atrial fibrillation. Stroke. Oral contraceptive pill, lymphoma, migraine.

EPIDEMIOLOGY Incidence <1/100 000 per year.

HISTORY Sudden profound, monocular loss of vision (central retinal artery occlusion) or altitudinal field of vision (branch retinal vein occlusion). Painless. Symptoms of causes, especially GCA, should be elicited. Some patients may have amaurosis fugax.

EXAMINATION Poor visual acuity. White retina. Cherry red spot at the macula. Cholesterol emboli (hollenhurt plaques) may be seen in retinal vessels in branch occlusion. Central vision can be preserved if a patient's retina features the anatomical variant of a patent cilioretinal artery. Carotid auscultation for bruit and cardiovascular examination to detect, for example an arrhythmia or valvular disease.

PATHOLOGY/PATHOGENESIS Most cases are due to the obstruction of blood flow to the retina by thrombosis within the central retinal artery or by cholesterol embolus. The choroid, whose blood supply is via the posterior ciliary arteries, supplies the fovea with oxygen and nutrients by diffusion independent of a blood supply from the retinal artery; hence the fovea appears to be unaffected. In constrast the remainder of the affected retina appears white because of oedema (axoplasmic stasis) in the superficial nerve fibre layer.

INVESTIGATIONS FBC, ESR, ECG, Blood glucose, lipids. Depending on suspicion of underlying causes; echocardiocraphy, carotid artery ultrasound, clotting screen, autoantibodies.

MANAGEMENT
• GCA should be treated urgently.
• *Urgent ophthalmological referral:* ocular massage, paracentesis of the anterior chamber, IV acetazolamide – may be attempted if within 48 hours of symptom onset.

COMPLICATIONS Permanent visual loss.

PROGNOSIS One-third patients with central retinal artery occlusion will not have any improvement in visual acuity. Branch occlusion has a better prognosis.

Retinal detachment ▶

DEFINITION Separation of the neurosensory rentina from the retinal pigment epithelium (RPE).

AETIOLOGY
- *Rhegmatogenous retinal detachment (RRD)*: retinal breaks/tears, macular holes.
- *Exudative retinal detachment (ERD)*: intraocular tumours, CMV retinitis, laser photocoagulation, malignant hypertension, eclampsia, Coat's disease.
- *Tractional retinal detachment (TRD)*: proliferative retinopathy.

ASSOCIATIONS/RISK FACTORS Myopia, cataract surgery, ocular/head trauma, diabetes mellitus.

EPIDEMIOLOGY Prevalence 0.3%.

HISTORY Photopsia, followed by showers of floaters and persistent visual field loss (curtain like, shadow/cloud/blurring). Check for history of trauma, surgery, diabetes and myopia.

EXAMINATION Visual acuity may be normal if the macula remains attached, Macular detachment causes severe visual loss. Visual field defect. RAPD (in extensive retinal detachment). Vitreous haemorrhage (may obscure view on fundoscopy).

PATHOLOGY/PATHOGENESIS
- *RRD:* a hole or tear develops in the retina. This may be due to predisposition, for example in myopia where the neurosensory retina is thinner and attached more weakly to the RPE. Degenerating vitreous can lead to excessive vitreoretinal or vitreomacular traction and precipitate a break. Following a break or tear in the retina, vitreous gel enters and separates the neurosensory retina from the RPE.
- *ERD:* there is fluid accumulation between the RPE and neurosensory retina that separates the layers. It does not enter through a tear or break in the retina.
- *TRD:* mechanical traction, caused for example by fibrovascular growth in proliferative diabetic retinopathy, causes detachment of the retina without a break or tear.

INVESTIGATIONS B-Scan ultrasound if there is impaired view of the fundus.

Retinal detachment ▶ (continued)

MANAGEMENT Urgent referral to an ophthalmologist. Various surgical and laser treatment modalities exist. These include laser photocoagulation, vitrectomy, scleral buckling, cyrotherapy and intraocular gas/oil tamponade.

COMPLICATIONS There is a risk of any retinal detachment to progress. Vitreous haemorrhage.

PROGNOSIS If the macula remains attached the visual prognosis following treatment is good. The contralateral eye is at risk of detachment. Poor prognosis is associated with macular detachment, especially if treatment is delayed.

Retinal vein occulsion ▶

DEFINITION Occlusion of the central retinal vein or a branch of it.

AETIOLOGY Age, hypertension, diabetes, hypercholesterolaemia.

ASSOCIATIONS/RISK FACTORS Raised intraocular pressure – increased risk of central retinal vein occlusion (CRVO).

EPIDEMIOLOGY Prevalence 4% in those over 80 years. Branch retinal vein occlusions (BRVO) are three times more common than CRVO.

HISTORY CRVO can be divided into ischaemic and nonischaemic types:

- *Nonischaemic CRVO:* painless, unilateral visual blurring.
- *Ischaemic CRVO:* sudden, painless (in most cases) and severe loss of vision.
- *BRVO:* can be ischaemic or nonischaemic but needs FFA to distinguish. More usefully classified based on the area of the fundus involved. May be symptomless but visual symptoms depend on the extent of the occlusion. Symptoms include sudden onset blurring or field defect.

EXAMINATION
- *Nonischaemic CRVO*: vision usually better than 6/60. Haemorrhages in all four quadrants. Possible RAPD.
- *Ischaemic CRVO:* RAPD. Widespread retinal haemorrhage in all four quadrants of the retina and cotton wool spots. Vitreous haemorrhage.
- *BRVO*: flame-shaped haemorrhages limited to the affected quadrant/region.

PATHOLOGY/PATHOGENESIS
- Thrombus occludes the central retinal vein at, or just posterior to, the lamina cribosa in CRVO.
- BRVO occurs at arteriovenous crossings where hardened atherosclerotic arterioles compress the vein, leading to turbulence of blood flow that leads to subsequent thrombus formation and obstruction.
- Retinal vein obstructions lead to a pressure build-up in the capillaries with resultant haemorrhage and fluid leakage. The effectiveness of blood perfusion is reduced and ischaemia can ensue.

INVESTIGATIONS Blood pressure, FBC, ESR, Blood glucose, U&Es, lipid profiles, thyroid function tests, plasma protein electrophoresis, ECG. Ischaemic and nonischaemic types can be differentiated based on FFA.

Retinal vein occulsion ▶ (continued)

MANAGEMENT Blood pressure control. Lifestyle adaptations including smoking cessation, weight loss and exercise. Laser photocoagulation, anti-VEGF agents and intraocular steroids are indicated in selected patients.

COMPLICATIONS Rubeosis (new vessel growth on the iris) and resultant glaucoma. Macular oedema. Painful eye.

PROGNOSIS Ischaemic CRVO has the worst prognosis with 40% progressing to rubeosis within 4 months.

Retinitis pigmentosa and other inherited retinal dystrophies

Retinitis pigmentosa

- This can be due to an inherited (autosomal dominant; 40% autosomal recessive 20%, X-linked) or sporadic mutation; 15% of cases are due to mutations in the rhodopsin gene. In the initial stages it causes progressive loss of rod photoreceptor function. This causes poor vision especially at night and loss of peripheral vision over time. Fundus examination reveals characteristic 'bone spicule' pigmentation, waxy pallor of the optic disc, and arteriolar narrowing. There may be associated cataracts.
- This condition has a poor visual prognosis in the long term and most patients will be registered as blind by the age of 40.

Albinism

- *Oculocutaneous albinism:* this is an autosomal recessive inherited condition characterized by melanin production defects. Patients will have very pale skin and white hair. It causes severe visual loss, photophobia and nystagmus. There will be absence of fundal pigmentation.
- *Ocular albinism:* hypomelanosis is confined to ocular structures. It can be X-linked or rarely autosomal recessive. Sufferers will have reduced visual acuity, nystagmus and hypopigmented fundi.

Leber congenital amaurosis

This is the commonest genetically inherited cause of visual impairment in infants. It has an autosomal recessive inheritance. Features include absent pupil reflexes and the eyes of sufferers may show roving movements. The fundus may be normal or there may be pigmentation of the macula or fundus and drusen at the optic disc. It has a very poor visual prognosis.

Stargardt's disease

Mostly inherited in an autosomal recessive pattern, this condition has a childhood onset and causes macular degeneration. Patients will have worsening central vision, for example when reading, by their 20s. They will suffer from profound visual loss by the age of 50 years. Signs of macular degeneration appear including yellow lipofuscin flecks around the macula.

Retinoblastoma ▶

DEFINITION Malignant intraocular tumour of infancy arising from primitive photoreceptor cells. Lethal if untreated.

AETIOLOGY
- Mutation of both alleles of the RB tumour-suppressor gene causes the development of retinoblastoma. In inherited cases, one mutation is inherited, and a second acquired mutation leads to deregulation of retinal cell growth.
- The increased susceptibility of all cells to deregulation is because there is one mutant copy of each allele in every cell because the first mutation was present in a germinal cell. Only one further mutation, to the normal allele, is therefore required to lose all function of the RB tumour suppressor gene.
- The detrimental acquisition of a second mutation in inherited cases, as described by Knudson in his 2-hit hypothesis, leads to the observation that inherited cases affect both eyes whereas sporadic cases are most often unilateral. This is because the chances of acquiring two mutations to a gene are much less than acquiring one mutation.

ASSOCIATIONS/RISK FACTORS The retinoblastoma gene is found to be deleted in patients with isolated osteosarcoma.

EPIDEMIOLOGY Prevalence: 1/20 000. 40% of cases are inherited.

HISTORY Leukocoria (white pupil reflex, may be noted by family on photographs). Strabismus, red eye. Orbital inflammation. Proptosis. Family history.

EXAMINATION Esotropia/exotropia. Raised intraocular pressure. Leukocoria on direct ophthalmoscope examination. White intraocular mass. Orbital examination and lymph node examination in cases of invasion. Raised intraocular pressure. General physical examination to check for metastasis.

PATHOLOGY/PATHOGENESIS
- Arises from retinal precursor cells.
- *Macro:* can appear as a white mass. May directly invade the vitreous, optic nerve or the subretinal space.
- *Micro:* high mitotic rates may manifest with varying differentiated forms of retinal cell structures; Homer-Wright rosettes, Flexner-Wintersteiner rosettes, fleurettes.

Retinoblastoma ▶ (continued)

INVESTIGATIONS Imaging – ocular ultrasound, magnetic resonance imaging of the orbit and skull. Bone scan. Lumbar puncture and bone marrow aspiration if metastatic disease. Genetic studies.

MANAGEMENT
- Depends on size of tumour.
- Chemotherapy, photocoagulation, cyrotherapy or focal radiation therapy for smaller tumours may be sufficient.
- Chemotherapy and enucleation for larger tumours.
- Treatment of metastasis if present.
- Family/genetic counselling and screening for prevention.

COMPLICATIONS Tumour spread to brain. Haematogenous metastatic dissemination to bone and viscera. Risk of second malignancy increases to 30% if external beam radiotherapy was used to treat the initial tumour.

PROGNOSIS Early diagnosis and treatment can lead to cure in over 90% of cases. There is a 6% risk of a second malignancy. Retinoblastoma is associated with increased risk of developing sarcoma and carcinoma. 3% of patients develop trilateral retinoblastoma which is bilateral retinoblastoma with a suprasellar primitive neuroectodermal tumour.

Retinopathy of prematurity (ROP) ▶

DEFINITION A proliferative retinopathy that affects premature infants given oxygen supplementation post-partum.

AETIOLOGY Vascularization of the retina is not complete until one month after the birth of a full-term neonate. Premature infants are exposed to relatively high concentrations of oxygen in the Paediatric intensive care units that they are being nursed in. The relative hyperoxia down-regulates vascular endothelial growth factor (VEGF) production which results in a poorly vascularized retina. On cessation of oxygen supplementation, the retina, because of incomplete vascularization, is hypoxic and this stimulates the release of VEGF. However, the subsequent vascularization is disorganized.

ASSOCIATIONS/RISK FACTORS Low birthweight (<1500 g), early gestational age (<32 weeks), High tension oxygen supplementation.

EPIDEMIOLOGY Was the leading cause of childhood blindness in the 1940s. Occurs in around 50% of those with the aforementioned risk factors.

HISTORY Obstetric history, birth weight and gestational age.

EXAMINATION Examine for a red reflex (can cause leukocoria), poor vision. Dilated indirect fundoscopy will be performed by an experienced ophthalmologist. Location and extent of disease can be determined and staging assessed.

PATHOLOGY/PATHOGENESIS Retinal vasculature develops from the hyaloid vessels at the optic disc and emanates peripherally during gestation. Vessels reach the nasal periphery of the retina by 32 weeks but do not reach the temporal periphery until 40 weeks. Following return of an infant to an environment of normal oxygen tension, the disorganized neovascular and fibrovascular growth can lead to retinal detachment and haemorrhage.

INVESTIGATIONS Retinal photography. Ultrasound.

MANAGEMENT
• Screening of neonates under 32 weeks gestation and of a weight less than 1500 g should be performed by ophthalmologists with specialist training in the condition.
• Monitoring in the less severe stages of the disease. Laser photocoagulation in selected cases.
• Surgery – indicated in severe cases where tractional retinal detachment has occurred.

Retinopathy of prematurity (ROP) ▶ (continued)

COMPLICATIONS Vitreous/retinal haemorrhage. The risks from examination and treatment (if under a GA) must be considered as the latter is associated with mortality.

PROGNOSIS Most cases of ROP will regress spontaneously. Early retinal detachment can be visually devastating. Some develop strabismus or amblyopia. Infants will be predisposed to retinal detachment and acute angle closure glaucoma in later life. Myopia and anisometropia is common.

Sarcoidosis (and Tuberculosis)

DEFINITION A chronic, multisystem inflammatory disorder characterized by the presence of noncaseating granuloms in affected tissues.

AETIOLOGY Unknown. A combination of genetic and environmental factors have been implicated. There is some evidence of association with HLA-B8.

ASSOCIATIONS/RISK FACTORS Unknown. There is limited evidence that industrial or agricultural dust exposure may increase the risk of developing sarcoidosis. There are reports of familial clustering of the disease.

EPIDEMIOLOGY UK incidence is 5/100 000. It can occur at any age but most commonly affects the young and middle aged. It is more common in Black people, who are also more severely affected, than Whites. It is more common in females.

HISTORY The disease may be asymptomatic and identified incidentally following routine chest X-ray. There may be fever, malaise or weight loss. Presentation can be acute for example with erythema nodosum and arthralgia. Chronic sarcoidosis can present with slowly progressive breathlessness due to pulmonary fibrosis. Otherwise, presentation depends on the system affected, therefore can be diverse.

OCULAR MANIFESTATIONS It has been suggested that ocular manifestations are only second to pulmonary features with regards to frequency. Anterior uveitis in patients normally has a subacute presentation with relatively few symptoms

EXAMINATION Positive findings depend on the system affected, for example:

- *Respiratory:* fine inspiratory crepitations due to pulmonary fibrosis.
- *Cardiovascular:* cardiac failure, pericarditis, conduction defects.
- *Joints:* terminal phalangeal bone cysts.
- *Neurological system:* cranial nerve palsies, space occupying lesions, peripheral neuropathy. Pituitary involvement can cause endocrine disturbance.
- *Abdominal:* hepatosplenomegaly.
- *Skin* : erythema nodosum, lupus pernio.
- *Head and neck:* parotid, salivary or lacrimal gland swelling.

Sarcoidosis (and Tuberculosis) (continued)

- *Ophthalmic*
  - Examination should include pupil reflexes, vision, colour vision, eye movements and fundoscopy.
  - Eye movement examination may reveal abnormality due to granuloma within the orbit or cranial nerve involvement. The former may be associated with proptosis.
  - *Anterior uveitis:* circumlimbal injection. The pupil may be irregular due to the formation of posterior synechaie. The cornea may appear cloudy and on slit lamp examination relatively large endothelial deposits will be apparent (mutton-fat keratic precipitates). There will be inflammatory activity in the anterior chamber (cells/flare). There may be nodules or granulomas apparent on the iris.
  - *Posterior uveitis:* ophthalmoscopy may reveal occlusion of vessels and perivascular exudation (this has been described as candle-wax dripping). Granulomatous nodules or atrophic spots may be observed on the fundus. There may be cystoid macular oedema (this is a common cause of poor vision in sarcoidosis).
  - *Optic nerve:* the optic nerve may be swollen due to papillitis, granulomatous infiltration or raised intracranial pressure secondary to an intracranial space occupying granuloma.
  - *Intermediate uveitis:* an ophthalmologist may observe vitritis on slit lamp examination.

PATHOLOGY/PATHOGENESIS Granulomas are localized collections of epitheloid macrophages; in sarcoidosis these do not undergo caseation necrosis. Granuloma formation can occur in response to an antigen however, in sarcoidosis it is unknown why such a reaction occurs. Multinucleate giant cells within granulomas contain inclusion bodies known as asteroid bodies and Schaumann bodies.

INVESTIGATIONS
- Raised serum angiotensin-converting enzyme (produced by the activated macrophages). Raised ESR, serum calcium. Reduced white cell count.
- *Chest X-ray:* bilateral hilar lymphadenopathy.
- *High resolution CT thorax:* to detect diffuse lung involvement if not apparent on chest X-ray
- *Head CT:* to help diagnosis neurosarcoidosis.
- *Biopsy:* of lesions may reveal features characteristic of granulomas.

Sarcoidosis (and Tuberculosis) (continued)

- *Lung function tests:* may reveal a restrictive picture.
- *Gallium67:* shows characteristic patterns of uptake in affected parotid or lacrimal glands.
- *Fundus fluorescein angiography:* to check for retinal ischaemia, new vessel formation or leaky vessels.

MANAGEMENT

- *Systemic:* slowly reducing prednisolone therapy is used for symptomatic cardiac, pulmonary or neurosarcoidosis. Nonsteroidal anti-inflammatory agents are used in less severe disease.
- *Ocular:* uveitis is treated with steroids by ophthalmologists. Topical steroid therapy is sufficient for most anterior segment inflammation. Posterior or intermediate uveitis may require intravitreal or systemic steroid use. Occasionally cytotoxic or immunomodulatory agents are required. Optic nerve involvement may require the use of pulsed intravenous steroids.

COMPLICATIONS

- Multiple organ involvement, death.
- *Ocular:* Cataract, glaucoma, chronic uveitis.

PROGNOSIS Most recover with no significant impairment (60% of those with thoracic sarcoid). Patients who do not respond to steroid therapy have a poorer prognosis.

Note on tuberculosis (TB)

TB is a multisystemic disease causes by *Mycobacterium tuberculosis*. It can present with similar features to sarcoidosis. Pulmonary involvement is the most common manifestation and classic features of the disease include cough, weight loss, night sweats and haemoptysis. The granulomos of TB feature caseating necrosis, in contrast to sarcoid granulomas. Ocular TB can cause a spectrum of ocular features that includes uveitis, vitritis, retinitis, retinal vessel occlusions, choroiditis and orbital abscesses. Emperic treatment of TB utilizes a combination of Rifampicin, Isoniazid, Pyrazinamide and Ethambutol.

Scleritis ▶

DEFINITION Inflammation of the sclera.

AETIOLOGY Idiopathic. 50% of cases are associated with an underlying systemic condition.

ASSOCIATIONS/RISK FACTORS
- Rheumatoid arthritis, systemic lupus erythematosis, gout, relapsing polychondritis, Wegener's granulomatosis, polyarteritis nodosa, giant cell arteritis, sero-negative arthropathy, sarcoidosis.
- Infectious agents such as TB, syphilis and varicella zoster may be associated with scleritis.
- Trauma or surgery can induce the condition.

EPIDEMIOLOGY Rare. More common in women. Peak incidence in those in their 50s.

HISTORY Eye pain: severe, deep, boring in nature. The pain disturbs sleep. It can radiate to the eyebrow, forehead or jaw. Exacerbated by eye movements. Minimal and temporary relief of pain from analgesics. Epiphora. Photophobia. Tender globe. Nausea/vomiting. Redness of the eye. Patients may complain of reduced vision. A detailed and expansive systemic history should be obtained.

EXAMINATION
- Systemic examination may reveal underlying disease.
- Reduced visual acuity.
- Examination in daylight – the sclera may appear red/blue. There will be injection of deep episcleral vessels that do not blanch on phenylephrinene (10% drop) instillation. There may be areas of scleral translucency (blue tinged) indicating thinning due to previous episodes of scleritis. A severe necrotizing form of scleritis would be indicated by black or brown areas. An area of central whiteness indicates that this area has become avascular.
- Slit lamp examination – corneal/intraocular inflammation. Thickened oedematous sclera.

PATHOLOGY/PATHOGENESIS
- *Diffuse/nodular, non-necrotizing scleritis:* nongranulomatous (initially) inflammation with scleral infiltrates of mononuclear cells. Granulomatous lesions can subsequently develop.
- *Necrotizing scleritis:* fibrinoid necrosis can occur and lead to scleral thinning. There is granulomatous inflammation around stromal collagen with T-cell and macrophage infiltration.

Scleritis ▶ (continued)

- *Scleratomalacia perforans* is a necrotizing form of scleritis without inflammation that is seen in rheumatoid arthritis. It is often asymptomatic in the initial stages but the eye is predisposed to perforation, for example with minor trauma.

INVESTIGATIONS FBC, U&Es with Uric acid, serum ACE, syphilis serology, ESR, CRP, rheumatoid factor, antinuclear antibody, antineutrophil cytoplasmic antibodies, double-stranded DNA. Chest X-ray. BP. Urine analysis (for casts). B-scan ocular ultrasound may reveal the rare condition 'posterior scleritis'.

MANAGEMENT
- Joint management between ophthalmologists and rheumatologists.
- Systemic NSAIDs, corticosteroids or immunosupression with agents such as azathioprine, cyclophosphamide or mycophenolate mofetil may be needed.
- There is some evidence supporting the use of Infliximab in refractory cases. Surgery may be needed to maintain the integrity of the globe in perforating cases.

COMPLICATIONS Scleral perforation, macular oedema, retinal detachment, glaucoma, uveitis, cataract.

PROGNOSIS Often benign in the absence of systemic disease. Necrotizing scleritis has a poor visual outcome.

Squint (strabismus), childhood

DEFINITION Misalignment of the visual axes. However, a squint may or may not be present at all times or in all different directions of gaze. See below.

AETIOLOGY Congenital/Idiopathic. Refractive error. Intracranial space occupying lesions. Cataract. Retinoblastoma may present with a squint.

ASSOCIATIONS/RISK FACTORS Cerebral palsy, Craniofacial abnormalities.

EPIDEMIOLOGY Up to 2% of children may have a squint.

HISTORY May be noted by parents/seen in photographs. There may be a history of varying or intermittent squint. It is important to elicit a history of a worsening or new squint as this may suggest sinister underlying pathology. There may be family history of squint.

EXAMINATION
- *Eye movements:* will help differentiate the following.
  - *Incomitant strabismus:* the angle of deviation would differ in different directions of gaze.
  - *Concomitant strabismus:* the angle of deviation is the same regardless of the direction of gaze.
- *Corneal light-reflex test:* a pen torch is held at a distance that causes a reflection of light to fall upon the corneas. The position of the reflections should be in the centre of each pupil. If not, a squint may be present.
- *Cover test:* the patient should be looking at a target. One eye is covered with an occluder. The uncovered eye is observed. If the uncovered eye moves to look at the target (i.e. takes up fixation), a manifest squint is present in that eye.
- *Uncover test:* one eye is covered and that eye is observed to check if it moves (to take up fixation) on removal of the cover. This would indicate a latent squint in that eye.
- These and other tests for squint can be difficult to interpret and are best performed by orthoptists in the setting of paediatric ophthalmology clinics.

PATHOLOGY/PATHOGENESIS
- *Concomitant (non-paralytic):* these are usually congenital and no diplopia will be present. The squint remains the same (i.e. the angle between the visual angle) in all directions of gaze.

Squint (strabismus), childhood (continued)

- *Incomitant (paralytic):* a rare form of squint due to a neurological defect of the motor nerve supply to the ocular muscles. It is normally acquired and may suggest an intracranial malignancy. If onset is in adulthood diplopia will be a feature and will be worse in the direction of action of the weak muscle. The angle between the axes of the eyes vary depending on direction of gaze. The image from the 'paralysed' eye will be on the 'outside' compared to the image from the normal eye.

INVESTIGATIONS Depend on suspected underlying causes.

MANAGEMENT
- All squints in children less than 9 years of age must be referred to prevent potential amblyopia and detect underlying refractive errors.
- *Correction of underlying causes:* glasses may be sufficient in appropriate cases.
- *Surgical:* corrective squint surgery may be performed in absence of sinister underlying causes and if the squint has been stable for at least 6 months.

COMPLICATIONS Amblyopia. Lack of binocular vision.

PROGNOSIS Correction at an early age is essential to prevent amblyopia.

Thyroid eye disease

DEFINITION An orbitopathy associated with thyroid dysfunction.

AETIOLOGY Mostly associated with Graves' disease.

ASSOCIATIONS/RISK FACTORS Female gender. Smoking, poor thyroid control, radioactive iodine treatment.

EPIDEMIOLOGY Women more frequently affected than men.

HISTORY Symptoms of thyroid disease should be ascertained as there may be active hyper or hypothyroidism. Symptoms of thyroid eye disease include: red eye, puffy eyelids, dry eyes, bulging eyes, diplopia, visual loss, pain/ache.

EXAMINATION
• Thyroid status should be assessed. Ocular signs of thyroid eye disease include conjunctival chemosis, proptosis, eye movement problems and diplopia. Lid lag and lid retraction are signs of the sympathomimetic hyperthyroid state in acute disease.
• In chronic disease, the signs can be due to proptosis and contraction of the upper eyelid retractor muscles.
• Compression of the optic nerve can lead to visual field loss and optic neuropathy with colour vision defect, a RAPD and pallor of the optic disc. There may be signs of corneal exposure.

PATHOLOGY/PATHOGENESIS Lymphocytes infiltrate the orbital connective tissue, fat and extraocular muscles. The cytokines released by lymphocytes stimulate fibroblasts to secrete connective tissue. Crowding of the 'closed box' like orbital compartment causes protrusion of the eye and potential optic nerve compression. Within 2 years of the active inflammation, fibrosis and scaring of the orbital contents ensues.

INVESTIGATIONS Thyroid function tests. MRI orbits - thickening of the ocular muscles.

MANAGEMENT
• Inadequately controlled thyroid disease should be managed. Smoking cessation must be emphasized. Artificial tears may help with dry eye. Eyelid surgery (e.g. tarsorraphy) may be required for exposure keratitis.
• High-dose steroids should be considered if there is optic nerve compression. Emergency surgical decompression may be indicated if there is no response. Orbital decompression surgery and eyelid correction can be attempted for cosmetic and functional reasons if thyroid eye disease had been stable for at least 6 months.

Thyroid eye disease (continued)

COMPLICATIONS Optic nerve compression. Exposure keratopathy.

PROGNOSIS Progressive disease results from inadequate treatment. The condition normally 'burns out' within 18 months without further recurrence.

Uveitis, anterior ▶

DEFINITION Inflammation of the iris and ciliary body.

AETIOLOGY Mostly idiopathic.

ASSOCIATIONS/RISK FACTORS HLA-B27. Ankylosing spondylitis, seronegative arthritis. inflammatory bowel disease, sarcoidosis, trauma, cataract surgery. Infectious causes – tuberculosis, syphilis. Herpes virus.

EPIDEMIOLOGY Annual incidence 8/100 000.

HISTORY Pain, photophobia, red eye. Blurred vision. Ask for symptoms of associated conditions.

EXAMINATION
- Circumcorneal/limbal injection, constricted pupil (may be irregular due to formation of posterior synechiae). Hypopyon.
- *Slit lamp:* endothelial corneal deposits, cells in the anterior chamber, flare.

PATHOLOGY/PATHOGENESIS There is T-cell and macrophage mediated inflammation. This is associated with breakdown of the blood-ocular barrier allowing extravasation of white blood cells and protein into the aqueous.

INVESTIGATIONS May not be needed in all cases. Target towards identifying underlying causes. Typically bilateral and recurrent cases require investigation.

MANAGEMENT Refer to ophthalmology; this condition cannot be diagnosed unless posterior uveitis has been excluded. Cycloplegic drops, such as cyclopentolate prevents formation of posterior synechiae and can relieve pain. Most cases respond to a tapering course of topical corticosteroids.

COMPLICATIONS Glaucoma, cataract, macular oedema, posterior synechiae, recurrence.

PROGNOSIS HLA-B27 associated disease is more prone to recurrence.

Uveitis, intermediate ▶

DEFINITION Inflammation of the vitreous, peripheral retina and ciliary body.

AETIOLOGY Most cases are idiopathic.

ASSOCIATIONS/RISK FACTORS
• Sarcoidosis, multiple sclerosis, inflammatory bowel disease, lymphoma.
• Infectious-HIV, Lyme disease, human T-cell lymphocyte virus type 1, toxacara, TB.

EPIDEMIOLOGY Rare, accounting for 5% of cases of uveitis.

HISTORY Floaters, blurred vision. Painless.

EXAMINATION The eye will not be red. Slit lamp examination will reveal cells in the vitreous; snow balls of inflammatory cell accumulations may be seen. Macular oedema may be apparent.

PATHOLOGY/PATHOGENESIS There is T-cell mediated inflammation of the vitreous.

INVESTIGATIONS May not be needed and if performed should be targeted towards clinically suspected causes.

MANAGEMENT The underlying condition should be treated if identified. Intra/periocular steroids may be effective. Surgical vitrectomy is indicated in some cases.

COMPLICATIONS Macular oedema, vitreous haemorrhage, glaucoma, retinal detachment.

PROGNOSIS 15% of patients with intermediate uveitis will develop multiple sclerosis. There is poor visual prognosis in severe disease that has affected the macula.

Uveitis, posterior ▶

DEFINITION Inflammation of the choroid and retina.

AETIOLOGY Idiopathic. Infectious causes are diverse and can be fungal, viral, bacterial, protozoal or nematode. Sympathetic ophthalmia.

ASSOCIATIONS/RISK FACTORS A diverse range of immunological conditions can be associated with this including sarcoidosis, Behçet's disease and vasculitis. Malignancy can masquerade as posterior uveitis.

EPIDEMIOLOGY This is very rare.

HISTORY Painless (However, can co-exist with anterior uveitis which is painful). Floaters, photopsia, blurred vision.

EXAMINATION Look for signs of systemic associations. Signs of anterior uveitis may be present. Regions of pallor and haemorrhage may be apparent on the retina. There may be papillitis. Cotton wool spots. Most other ocular changes will require slit lamp examination.

PATHOLOGY/PATHOGENESIS There is an immune response, involving T-cells and monocytes, directed at uveal peptides. Sympathetic ophthalmia involves an insult, usually traumatic, that allows immune exposure and subsequent T-cell mediated response to a previously immune privileged ocular antigen. The response is bilateral despite uniocular insult.

INVESTIGATIONS Syphilis serology is essential. Other investigations should be targeted towards identifying possible underlying causes based on clinical suspicion in the first instance and excluding other treatable infectious causes.

MANAGEMENT Ophthalmologists will normally make this diagnosis. Management is conservative in mild cases where vision is unaffected. Immunosuppression and targeted therapy towards the underlying causes.

COMPLICATIONS This can be sight threatening. Retinal detachment, glaucoma, macular/optic disc infarction can occur.

PROGNOSIS 50% of cases will retain good vision.

Glossary

Accomodation reflex   Fixation on near object causes convergence, miosis and increased convexity of the lens.

Anti-vascular endothelial growth factor (anti-VEGF)   Agents that block the effects of vascular endothelial growth factor.

Amsler grids   A series of grids designed to record distortion/blurring or field defects of central (macular) vision. Patients are asked to look at the centre of the grid and then either explain, or draw on to a recording grid, any of the aforementioned defects.

Anisocoria   Difference in size of pupil – there is a physiological difference of up to 2 mm in pupil size.

Anisometropia   Difference in refractive error between eyes.

Chemosis   Oedema of the conjunctiva.

Cicatricial   Describes scarring formed by deposition of connective tissue.

Conjunctival follicles   Discrete, elevated whitish/yellow coloured conjunctival lesions representing lymphoid collections.

Cycloplegic drugs   Pharmacological agents that can cause pupil dilation.

Cystoid macular oedema   Oedema of the macula with cyst formation, caused, for example, after cataract surgery.

Drusen   Yellow chorioretinal spots, may be well defined (hard) or larger and poorly defined (soft drusen).

Endophthalmitis   Inflammation of the intraocular structures; usually used to refer to inflammation caused by microbial contamination within the eye.

Epiphora   Excessive lacrimation/tearing; a watery eye.

Esotropia   A manifest deviation in which the the eye is turned inwards (medially).

Excyclotorsion   Outward rotation of the eye.

Exophthalmos   Protrusion of the eye. Sometimes this term is reserved for bilateral proptosis or proptosis due to thyroid eye disease.

Exotropia   A manifest deviation in which the eye is turned outwards (laterally).

Hypertropia   A manifest deviation where the affected eye gazes upwards; the visual axis of the affected eye is higher than the eye that is fixating.

Intorsion   Inward rotation of the eye.

Rapid Ophthalmology, First Edition. Zahir Mirza.
© 2013 John Wiley & Sons, Ltd. Published 2013 by John Wiley & Sons, Ltd.

Lagophthalmos   Inability to fully close the eye.
Latent squint/deviation or heterophoria   The eyes' visual axes are aligned when binocularly fixing on a target but deviate when the eyes are dissociated, for example, when performing the alternate cover test.
Leukocoria   White pupil.
Manifest squint/deviation or heterotropia   The affected eye's visual axis is not directed towards a fixation point.
Metamorphopsia   Visual distortion of shapes/objects.
Miosis   Constricted pupil.
Orthoptic   Relating to the measurement of eye-movements and the nonsurgical management of eye-movement disorders.
Papillae   These conjunctival lesions can range in appearance from red dots (due to a central vessel) to giant (cobblestone) papillae as multiple lesions coalesce.
Papillitis   Inflammation of the optic nerve head. Typically unilateral.
Papilloedema   Swelling of the optic nerve head due to raised intracranial pressure. Almost nearly always bilateral.
Photophobia   Sensitivity/aversion to light.
Proptosis   Outward protrusion of the eye.
Relative afferent pupillary defect (RAPD)   Following direct stimulation of a pupil by light, both pupils constrict in normal eyes. In the presence of a relative afferent papillary defect the following sequence would be observed.

1. Light shone on the normal pupil – constriction of both pupils.
2. Light then swung on to abnormal pupil – dilation of the (abnormal) pupil onto which the light is being shone (and simultaneous dilatation of the normal pupil).

A RAPD indicates a reduction in the afferent input from the retina of the abnormal eye compared to the normal eye because of an optic nerve defect in the former.
Sympathetic ophthalmia   A bilateral granulomatous uveitis that is very rare and occurs after surgery or trauma to one eye.
Trichiasis   In-turning eyelashes.

Index

Rapid Ophthalmology, First Edition. Zahir Mirza.
© 2013 John Wiley & Sons, Ltd. Published 2013 by John Wiley & Sons, Ltd.